Intended Parents: Miracles Do Happen

Intended Parents: Miracles Do Happen

✦

A True-Life Success Story of Having Children through Surrogacy

Sandra Watson Rapley

iUniverse, Inc.
New York Lincoln Shanghai

Intended Parents: Miracles Do Happen
A True-Life Success Story of Having Children through Surrogacy

Copyright © 2005 by Sandra Watson Rapley

All rights reserved. No part of this book may be used or reproduced by any means, graphic, electronic, or mechanical, including photocopying, recording, taping or by any information storage retrieval system without the written permission of the publisher except in the case of brief quotations embodied in critical articles and reviews.

iUniverse books may be ordered through booksellers or by contacting:

iUniverse
2021 Pine Lake Road, Suite 100
Lincoln, NE 68512
www.iuniverse.com
1-800-Authors (1-800-288-4677)

ISBN-13: 978-0-595-35528-0 (pbk)
ISBN-13: 978-0-595-80012-4 (ebk)
ISBN-10: 0-595-35528-5 (pbk)
ISBN-10: 0-595-80012-2 (ebk)

Printed in the United States of America

This book is dedicated to Craig, Jamie, Luke, Victoria, Clive, Marcus, and Chloe.

Contents

Introduction 1

Part I   The Discovery of Infertility
CHAPTER 1   The Betrayal 5
CHAPTER 2   The Offer 10
CHAPTER 3   More Fibroids! 13

Part II   Starting Our Journey
CHAPTER 4   Surrogacy Administrivia 17
CHAPTER 5   We Are Ready to Get Pregnant 24

Part III   Egg Retrieval and Transfer
CHAPTER 6   First Trimester 29
CHAPTER 7   We Are Pregnant! 35

Part IV   Our Pregnancy
CHAPTER 8   Twins! 41
CHAPTER 9   When Do I Tell People? 45
CHAPTER 10   Worry, Worry, Worry 47
CHAPTER 11   Second Trimester 55
CHAPTER 12   Meeting with the Genetic Counselor 60

Chapter 13	I Am Going to Be a Mommy!	64
Chapter 14	Third Trimester	69

Part V   The Birth of Our Boys

Chapter 15	Our Boys Finally Arrive!.	77

Part VI   Going Home

Chapter 16	Our Journey Home	87
Chapter 17	Family Life.	89

Part VII   Update

Chapter 18	Our Boys Today.	95

Afterword 97

Acknowledgments

I received a lot of support and encouragement from family and friends while I was writing this book. There are some people that I need to thank in particular, because without them this book would not have been written.

Thank you

To my husband Craig for your continued love, support, strength, friendship, encouragement, and sense of humor.

To my sons Jamie and Luke for coming into our lives and allowing Craig and me to love and guide you. We really wanted you both and we will be eternally grateful to you for allowing us to share your lives.

To Victoria, Clive, Marcus, and Chloe. From the bottom of my heart, thank you for deciding, as a family, that you wanted to make our dreams come true. Victoria, we will always be forever grateful to you.

To Fiona Kontou for allowing me to share my thoughts and feelings, even at my most stressful and crazy times. Thank you for always being there.

To Dr. Joel Batzofin for your skill, expertise, kindness, and compassion. You truly are a miracle worker.

And thanks also to Charles Watson, Sonia Messam, Charlene Messam, Andre Hadjioannou, Brenda Sobel, Hannah Caplan and Mia Whitman.

Introduction

My husband Craig and I were healthy, strong, financially stable, and ready to have children. It came as a big surprise when I found out that I couldn't have children. I knew that I would have some difficulty after surgeries I'd had, but I thought it would be just a simple matter of having some tests and perhaps some medical intervention and that would be that. Not so at all.

After having numerous tests and being subjected to multiple doctors' appointments and more questionnaires about my gynecological history, it soon became clear that I could not have children. This was a very hard pill to swallow. Wasn't it my right as a woman?

Surrogacy was our only option, and thanks to the generosity of my brother and sister-in-law, we finally realized our dream of having our family.

Before, during, and even after the process of surrogacy, I found that I was looking for someone or something to tell me that the feelings I was having were quite normal and okay. I wanted to be in sister-in-law Victoria's presence all the time. Was I crazy to feel this way? No one around me could answer this question, and I could not find the answer in any book I read. It wasn't a subject that you could discuss with just anybody.

For that reason I decided to write this book. *Intended Parents: Miracles Do Happen* looks at the emotional aspects of surrogacy and legitimizes those thoughts and feelings you have and are not able to share.

I share my thoughts and feelings with you, week by week, throughout our journey to finally bringing home our precious boys.

PART I
The Discovery of Infertility

1

The Betrayal

How could my body betray me this way? Here I was, thirty-nine years old, and I had just discovered that I couldn't have children. Why couldn't I have found this out when I was much younger? After all the years of trying not to get pregnant, I probably would not have become pregnant anyway! The hard part of all this was constantly hearing that never-ending sound of tick tock, tick tock! It seemed that I was always being asked when I was going to have children. After all, I *was* married and I *was* in my late thirties.

Every time someone asked this of me I felt the pain in my heart and the emptiness in the pit of my stomach. I tried to put on a brave face and smile while I was crying inside. How could they know that the questions they asked were so hurtful?

In 1987, I had the most painful period pains, with very heavy bleeding and large clots. I also had acute pains on the lower right side of my abdomen. I was rushed to the emergency room because my doctor thought I had appendicitis. After many tests, a sonogram revealed that I had large fibroids which were causing me a great deal of pain. Fibroids, also known as myomas, are non-cancerous growths which are masses of fibrous and muscle tissue in the uterine wall. Fibroids can cause heavy menstrual bleeding and pain in the pelvic region.

My doctor informed me that I would have to have a myomectomy which is a procedure where uterine fibroids are surgically removed from the uterus. At the post-operative consultation, the doctor said that I really ought to consider getting pregnant very soon. Well, I was horrified at the suggestion. I didn't even have a boyfriend! How could I consider having a child?

In 1995, I had a very painful period with heavy clotting again. I suspected that fibroids were causing the problem and a sonogram confirmed the diagnosis. Again I underwent a myomectomy to remove the fibroids. This post-operative consultation revealed that one of my fallopian tubes was surrounded by scar tissue from the previous surgery. The doctor said that many women had gone on to have babies after fibroid surgery and having only one tube. She also said that I really should think about having a family. I had a boyfriend this time, but I was just not ready for a child. I hung on to the fact that I had one fallopian tube and thought that it would work beautifully for me when the time came.

Over the years I would have a recurring dream about being pregnant. The funny thing about the dream was that each time I had it I would be a little further along in the "pregnancy" than the last time I had the dream. Consciously, I never thought about being pregnant. In fact, whenever anyone mentioned the word *children* to me I would scoff at the idea and say that I was too young. I guess I must have thought about it subconsciously, however, and that was why I had the occasional dream about it.

I met Craig in 1993, and we dated for five years before we got married in 1998. We decided to start having children straightaway. I was thirty-seven and Craig was thirty-eight. Each month I would go out and buy a pregnancy test kit and wonder if I were pregnant. I would imagine that I was pregnant because I had decided to have something different for breakfast that day, or I felt twinges in my abdomen. I would test and wait for a few minutes—and there would be nothing. I would try it again with a different brand. *Maybe there was something wrong with the first test,* I thought. *Surely the second one would show positive.*

After six months of peeing on sticks and slumping into the acceptance of not being pregnant—again—I decided that it was time to see my gynecologist. She prescribed Clomid to help me to ovulate and told me that I should start to check for ovulation from day 10 of my cycle. *All was not lost,* I thought. *These pills would correct the "problem" I had, and I would become pregnant soon. It worked for my friend Fiona, so why wouldn't it work for me?* I bought the ovulation kit as the doctor suggested and followed the instructions. I would diligently check each day as I was told to, and I found that I did not ovulate on day 10, 11, 12, 13, 14, 15, or day 16. No surprises there, I thought, because I only had one tube. Next month I would ovulate.

Meanwhile I noticed that I had no patience with anyone, especially Craig, my husband. I knew I was being very short with him, but I had no control over it. I was constantly picking at him for the slightest thing he said or did. He just took it in his stride, and that would make me even angrier with him. It was the strangest thing. I just could not control it. Eventually, after I stopped taking the drug, I realized that it must have been my reaction to Clomid.

The next month I checked for my ovulation from day 10 of my cycle, as prescribed by my doctor. I didn't ovulate. I checked again the following month, and I couldn't believe it. I did not ovulate. *How could this be? I have one good tube.*

Why wasn't it working? The first feelings of a long chain of helplessness started to kick in. I would remind myself that I knew it would be a bit more difficult because of the surgeries that I'd had. My head knew this, but my heart would not accept it. By day 13 I would become anxious, and by day 16 I would be devastated. I really was going to have a problem conceiving. I would feel so weak that all I could do was go to bed.

My friend Fiona told me about an ovulation kit called Clearblue Easy Fertility Monitor, where you test every day and it stores your results in memory. She suggested that perhaps I was ovulating, but at a different time than expected. The kit wasn't cheap, but I decided that I would buy it and see if there was a difference. There are three readings on this kit: low, medium, and high. The first 11 days of testing registered a low reading. Days 12 through 16 registered a medium reading. On day 17 I was bowled over with shock and surprise, because the reading was high! I was in shock because I had only tested up to day 16 in the prior three months! At last! I was over the moon and filled with hope. I do ovulate!

Running to Craig with the proof of ovulation, I told him that it was time to have sex. A couple of weeks later I would be disappointed again, with yet another negative pregnancy test followed rapidly by my period.

I continued to monitor my ovulation with the kit for another four months, and each month I ovulated on day 17. I would test for pregnancy, and again I would not be pregnant. I went back to my gynecologist, who said it was time for me to be seen by a specialist—a reproductive endocrinologist (RE). I had never heard of such a doctor.

A reproductive endocrinologist is an obstetrician-gynecologist (OB/GYN) who has advanced education and professional skills in reproductive endocrinology and infertility. I was a bit daunted at first. Reproductive endocrinologist—it was such a long title. What exactly did they do? I searched for reproductive endocrinology on the Internet and found that an RE provides diagnostic, medical, and surgical treatment, as well as laboratory services, for a wide variety of reproductive disorders. I was hopeful. Now that I was going to see a specialist, my problem would be identified and soon be resolved. I started to feel better about going to see yet another doctor.

After the appointment with my gynecologist, I went back to my office and contacted my medical insurance company to see if they had any recommendations for a specialist. They would not recommend anyone to me, but they would tell me which specialists were in my plan. While talking to them I found out that they would pay for everything to find out the cause of my not getting pregnant, but if in vitro fertilization (IVF) turned out to be a recommendation they would not pay for it. How could this be? *You will pay for everything to find out what the problem is, but you won't pay for the solution! What kind of plan was this?* I was dumbfounded.

This whole situation was getting more and more frustrating. *Sandra, you're jumping ahead again. Go to see the specialist. It might not be as complicated as you think.* I tried to reassure myself by thinking, *one step at a time.*

The insurance company gave me three names. I called all three. The first two doctors' next appointments were six months away. *Six months! I can't wait that long.* The third doctor's next appointment was three months away. I made an appointment for October 13, 1999. *How come the appointments are so far into the future? Maybe there are quite a few people out there who have similar problems to mine?*

The examination with the RE was typical. I had to fill out paperwork with lots of questions about my health and past surgeries. I then had an exam that was much the same as I'd had with my gynecologist. My RE then scheduled me for a hysterosalpingogram, an endometrial biopsy, and also a laparoscopy.

The hysterosalpingogram was done to see if my tubes were open. A dye was injected into my uterine cavity through the vagina and cervix. The uterine cavity was then filled with the dye, and the idea was that my fallopian tubes would also fill and the dye would then spill into my abdominal cavity. But my fallopian tubes did not fill and spill into the abdominal cavity. One tube was completely blocked, and the other tube just trickled a little dye.

The endometrial biopsy is a procedure that removes a small sample of the lining of the uterus that is examined under a microscope for abnormal cells. No abnormal cells were found, thankfully.

The laparoscopy is a procedure performed under general anesthetic that involves insertion of a narrow, telescope-like instrument through a small incision in the belly button. This procedure can identify abnormalities of the uterus, ovaries, and fallopian tubes. The procedure confirmed that both of my tubes had scar tissue from the two myomectomy surgeries I'd had. *No wonder I couldn't get pregnant; the egg couldn't get through.* Finally I was encouraged, because we had found out what the problem was.

At the post-operative consultation after the laparoscopy, our RE told us that our next step was IVF. At last we had a solution. I wanted to start the IVF procedures as soon as possible.

At this time I was working as a consultant for an information technology company, and they had just announced that they would give medical insurance to their consultants at the discounted group rate. I received the information packet they sent to me, found out the name of the insurance company, and contacted them to find out what coverage they offered for infertility. I could not believe it when the person I spoke to said they would cover up to $25,000 for infertility expenses. This included IVF treatments and medication. I could not believe it, so I called the company two more times and spoke to two different people who said the exact same thing. IVF treatment and medication were covered, so I joined the plan immediately. What good timing!

2

The Offer

Craig and I tried very hard to take our minds off being pregnant, so we had big round planters built in our back garden and filled them with butterfly bushes, lilies, daffodils, tulips, myrtle, and every other type of flowering plant we could fit in. This eased our minds a little bit, but we still pictured children running around them in the summer time. *How do you take your mind off something you are consumed with?* I decided not to bother to answer that question. I wanted to have children, and that was that.

When we started the IVF process, we told our friends we were doing it. When the results were negative, we found it really difficult when they would ask what was happening. I guess the real question was "were we pregnant"? They all meant well, but it was painful nonetheless. I started to avoid people so that I would not have to talk about it. I also started to not return phone calls, and I did not go out and meet up with my friends on a regular basis, as I used to. I found that I was consumed with babies and could think of nothing else, so instead of letting it slip, I avoided contact.

During the process of our IVF treatments there would be times when I felt so desperate and vulnerable. I would be self-confident before I had an appointment with our specialist, but then when I got there it was like I had lost all my courage. I felt that my doctor was always rushed. Even when I armed myself with questions I had written down and went through them one by one, she would still rush through. I decided to continue with her mainly because I did not want to wait six months for an appointment with another specialist.

In the summer of 2000 I was invited to a neighbor's baby shower. She was due in November, and I had calculated that if the first IVF treatment had been successful I would have been due in December. When I looked at her and saw how radiant she was, I kept thinking of myself and how radiant I would have been. I decided that I would go to the shower—why, I don't know.

The affair was set outside in their back garden, and there were a lot of people. Again, I was asked when I was going to have children. What did I expect? It was a baby shower, after all. I started to wonder what possessed me to go in the first place. While I was sitting there watching the gifts being opened, I felt a wave of tears coming over me. My body started to shake as if I were about to explode. I had to leave immediately. I told my neighbors that I had to go home and that I would be back shortly. I didn't go back, of course. How could I? I walked slowly back to my house. I felt that I was carrying a very heavy burden of pain on my shoulders as the tears streamed down my face.

I had kept in very close contact with my brother Clive during all of our procedures. He was very encouraging throughout, and forever the optimist. He would try to calm me down. I was anxious about all the procedures and while waiting for the results. There was absolutely nothing that would calm me down. I tried to relax, but I knew that all efforts would be futile, so I decided to accept that I would be worried about everything.

After the first IVF procedure failed, my brother told me that he had been talking to his wife Victoria and his children. They all agreed that if IVF didn't work for us, Victoria would be our surrogate mother and, hopefully, deliver a baby for us. I was in shock. Would someone really do this for someone else?

I had stumbled across the word *surrogacy* while researching IVF, but I never thought any more about it. At that time I still hoped that I would be able to get pregnant and deliver my own child. I kept on asking Clive over and over again whether Victoria really said yes. I even said that I hoped he was not joking around, because this really was no joking matter. He told me to call Victoria and ask her for myself. So I did.

I called her. She confirmed that their offer was real and true. I kept on asking her if she knew what would be involved—the many injections in the bottom, and going to the doctor on multiple occasions. She said she knew exactly what was involved, and she really wanted to do it for us. She said that she felt we really deserved to have a family, and if we couldn't do it on our own, then she would act as an "oven" for us. She would be just the carrier.

I was in a daze. This would be the greatest gift one person could ever give to another. Would they really do this for us? I called Craig immediately and told him what they'd said. "Can it be done?" he asked. I told him that I had stumbled across the word *surrogacy* on the Internet and found that many women were being surrogate mothers for infertile couples, even for people they did not know. I explained that the eggs would be retrieved from my ovaries as they had been in the past, during the IVF process. They would then be fertilized with his sperm and the embryos transferred to Victoria's uterus. He thought it was a fantastic offer and said that we should seriously think about it.

I started looking into surrogacy in a frenzy, and of course came across the Baby M case. This case was not a good advertisement for surrogacy, but I soon discovered that there were many successful surrogacy arrangements that were not being reported in the media. After I had time to calm down a bit, I called Victoria again to ask her if she really understood what would be involved. She said she, too, had been researching on the Internet and knew exactly what she would have to do. She kept telling me that she wanted to do it for us.

After the second IVF procedure failed we sank even lower than I ever thought possible. *How can this be? Yes, I knew I would have problems—but not this.* I wanted to spend most of my time in bed. It was so difficult to get out of bed and go to work when all I wanted to do was stay at home and cry. I was glad we had a routine. We had to go to work—that kept us going. Sometimes I would end up at home after a day at work and not remember how I got there.

My friends would arrange to get together for dinner and I just could not face them. I hadn't told them about the second IVF attempt, and I feared that they would be able to see it written all over my face.

Everywhere I turned there was nothing but babies—babies on television, babies in the supermarket, and babies in the street. I would look around and see families with infants, and I would feel very, very sad. Not only did I have the stress of not having a child when I wanted one, but I also had age against me. *Why us?* By this time, "why us" was like an old record that was constantly playing in my head.

I was still being asked when we were going to have children. How we managed to keep it together I will never know. We must have been in autopilot mode.

One day, a very nice woman at work came to my office and told me she was pregnant with twins. I don't think she noticed, but I was speechless. In the process of sitting down in my chair and looking down at the floor, I think I must have managed to put a smile on my face. This was the last thing I wanted or expected to hear. It took all my might to hold back the explosion that I felt inside of me. My throat was dry, and I felt that I would have trouble breathing. While she was talking to me I started to take deep breaths. I wasn't about to tell her that I desperately wanted a baby. Why should I? Eventually I reached a certain level of calmness and was able to utter a few words of congratulations. Clearly, she could not see my hands wringing together under my desk. By now I had learned to put on a brave front. I tried my hardest to sound happy for her, and I truly was happy for her. I was just very sad for myself. How I managed not to break down there and then I will never know. After she left my office I closed my door. I put my head in my hands and just cried and cried.

3

More Fibroids!

My husband was very supportive. He would try to comfort me and suggested that we should take Victoria and Clive up on their offer. He was more practical than I was. It was different for him, because he wasn't struggling with the age factor and the body-not-working-properly factor. I really felt that I was alone until my husband found some on-line mailing lists that were all about IVF, and joined them on my behalf. There were many women who were going through IVF. I befriended one woman in particular who was going through her treatment at the same time I was. We madly sent private messages to each other about how we were feeling, and about our thoughts and our dreams. Finally I had someone to share my thoughts with. At last!

A few days after the second transfer, I felt exactly the same as I did after the first transfer—the one that failed. My friend was trying to be encouraging to me, while telling me that she felt minor body changes like her breasts being a little tender. She wondered whether it was her period coming. We were both down in the dumps when we went in for our pregnancy tests. Later that day, the inevitable was confirmed for me. I sent her a private message and told her that my result was negative. She sent me a very happy message back, telling me that her result was positive. I couldn't stand it. The pain was unbearable. I wished her success and just switched off the computer. I could not and would not correspond with her again. I was happy for her, but I was very sad for myself—again.

We went to the doctor to discuss the negative results of our second IVF attempt. The doctor said she could see no reason why IVF would not work for us, and she started talking about doing another IVF attempt. Three times and no pregnancy would have been too much to bear. I insisted that there must be other tests we could do. She finally sent me for a pelvic sonogram which found fibroids. There were many fibroids in my uterus. I was in complete shock. The RE had told us about a fibroid on the outside of my uterus, but she never, ever told us about the many fibroids *inside* my uterus. *How could she not have seen them?* We'd had so many sonograms that I couldn't believe that she hadn't told us about this very important detail. When we went in to discuss the results, she just brushed us off. We tried to pin her down and asked her for an explanation as to why she did not tell us about the fibroids, and she kept on insisting that she did. How could we get pregnant with all those fibroids? She was very dismissive, and I started to wish that we had gone to another doctor.

I felt deflated. I didn't have the will or the strength to argue with her. All that time, money, and effort were all for naught. I felt that there was only one direction for us, and that was further down into the pits of depression. I just could not see myself without a baby. I wanted my own baby so badly. I left work early that day, went home, and went straight to bed. I knew that we should have found a new doctor, but we didn't want to wait six months for an appointment. Well, guess what. We had just wasted six months!

I was very cross with the doctor and very cross with my body. How could my body betray me like this? Why did I have to find out now when I was thirty-nine? I guess I should have paid more attention to the doctors when, after both surgeries, they were gently telling me that I should start thinking about having children. But how could I have children then? I wasn't ready then—but I was certainly ready now.

I spent the rest of the summer in a daze of trying to accept that my body didn't work in the way that I thought it should. Wasn't it my right as a woman to bear children? I found it a very hard pill to swallow. Meanwhile, everywhere I looked I saw babies and very young children. I found that I didn't suffer as much when I saw older children. I suffered the most when I saw babies and young children under the age of five.

PART II
Starting Our Journey

4

Surrogacy Administrivia

I kept on searching for surrogacy on the Internet, looking for experiences of other intended parents. I wanted to talk to someone who was sharing the same pain as I was. One of the first things I noticed was that there was not a lot of information from the intended parents' point of view. I searched for hours and days, and I couldn't find anything. There were plenty of surrogate mother stories, which I found refreshing, but I still wanted to find intended parents stories. I wanted to find intended mothers and ask them how they felt about the fact that they could not carry a child. I couldn't find anything.

Meanwhile, I was grieving. I was grieving because I knew that I would not be able to carry and deliver my own baby. Even though Victoria had kindly offered to be our surrogate mother, I couldn't accept her offer straight away because I had to get over the fact that I couldn't carry my own child. I still hoped that I would become pregnant. After a couple of months, I slowly came to the realization that this would not happen.

Throughout the summer I had contacted Victoria on various occasions to question her further and basically give her the opportunity to back out of her offer if she wanted to, but she never did. Finally, my brother Clive called to tell me to stop calling Victoria to talk her out of it. "We want to do this for you," he said very sternly. That confirmed it for me.

During this time I would have very vivid dreams about being pregnant, and again I would be a little further along in the "pregnancy" with each dream. Finally I dreamed that I was almost nine months pregnant, and feeling very uncomfortable. In this dream I was taken to the hospital and admitted to the labor and delivery ward. I was lying in the bed with many people surrounding me, and I was panting heavily, with my knees pulled up to my chest, as I was about to give birth. Everyone in the room was counting to ten in unison and telling me to push. My husband Craig was at my bedside, cheering me on. One final push and I heard the beautiful sound of a baby screaming. Everyone around me had beaming smiles, and I had tears of joy streaming down my face. I had just given birth to my long-awaited baby. The nurses swaddled my baby and handed him to me. My husband and I kept on kissing our baby and saying that we had waited so long for his arrival. There wasn't a dry eye in the room.

When I awoke from this dream I felt a sense of calm and acceptance. *I am going to have a baby.* As I went to work that day, I could still hear the sounds of my baby's cries ringing in my ears. It felt so real. Was I really going to have a baby?

I decided not to grieve anymore. The dream had given me a new sense of hope, and hope was what I desperately needed. Craig kept reminding me of Clive and Victoria's offer, and then I finally realized that there was a light at the end of the tunnel. I truly believed that we would have our baby, and I didn't have any more time to waste.

We contacted Clive and Victoria and told them that we would take them up on their extremely generous offer.

I started searching for information with a frenzy that I didn't know I possessed. I think that because I knew this would probably be our one and only chance of having a child, I threw my heart and soul into it. I wanted to know as much as I could about surrogacy, and as quickly as possible. Eventually I found out that California was the most surrogacy-friendly state, and Clive and Victoria lived in California. I found out that the type of surrogacy we wanted to do was gestational surrogacy, where my eggs and Craig's sperm would be used to create our embryos.

Where do we start? I decided to look for a fertility center in California. There were so many of them. How would I choose one over the other? This was an incredibly daunting task. Who would I ask for a reference? I didn't know anyone in my situation. I called a few centers and asked them to send information to me. Even after I received information, I still could not make a choice. After a number of days, I decided to see if any of the major hospitals in New York City had affiliations with any fertility centers in California. I knew that Cornell Hospital was well-known and well-respected, and I decided to start with them.

I searched Cornell's Web site and eventually found a link to a fertility center in Pasadena, California. As luck would have it, the fertility center was only about forty miles from where my brother and his family lived. I called the fertility center to see if they participated in surrogacy arrangements, and fortunately they did. I decided that we would work with them because, after all, if they were on the venerable Cornell Hospital's Web site, they must be good!

The first thing I decided to do was to get my medical records from my reproductive endocrinologist. Fortunately, they were able to provide me with them the same day. Once I picked them up, I took them back to work with me and made a copy. I was really surprised that my records were about two inches thick. This time I was not going to make the same mistake again. If either Victoria or I was uncomfortable with the doctor, I would look for another doctor immediately. This was too big a venture to feel uncomfortable with an important member of our "team".

Craig and I became the administrators of our pregnancy. We organized everything ourselves. It was a very strange concept to grasp, but we adapted to our roles very quickly.

I made appointments for Victoria and for myself at our new fertility center. Our appointment was with the esteemed Dr. Joel Batzofin, who was the medical director of the center. I was happy because there was a group of doctors in this practice, and we were going to have our appointments with the head of the center. We had to wait five weeks for an appointment, but at least it wasn't as bad as having to wait for three months!

Victoria had her appointment first. The doctor reviewed her medical records and examined her. She was given a hysteroscopy examination to make sure that her uterus looked normal. Victoria's blood was drawn to check for any sexually transmitted diseases. She was then given a referral for a mammogram. Victoria called and told me about the examination. She seemed to like the doctor and said everyone at the fertility center was very friendly. While she was in the waiting room a surrogate mother and an intended mother were waiting for their appointment. Victoria was happy to see that she was not alone.

At a separate time, my brother went to the fertility center to have his blood drawn, to check for sexually transmitted diseases.

My interview with the doctor was over the telephone, because we live in New Jersey. I had already sent my medical records to the fertility center in advance of my appointment. We discussed my medical history and also my reproductive history. The doctor reviewed the notes of my surgeries, other tests that I'd had, and also my IVF procedures. We discussed my previous IVF treatments, and we agreed that I would use the same protocol as I used with my IVF treatments because it had actually worked—I produced eggs. I decided that I liked Dr. Batzofin. I felt very comfortable with him, and he seemed to have all the time in the world. Not once did I feel rushed. After the telephone appointment I felt comfortable, but anxious—comfortable with the appointment, but anxious about surrogacy. *Were we crazy to even contemplate such a thing?* No, because at this point I truly believed I would do anything to have a baby.

The administrator at the fertility center stated clearly that before we could start working with them they would need clearance letters from our lawyer and our psychologist. The legal clearance letter would basically state that we had a contract with Victoria, our surrogate mother, which had been reviewed by her, her husband Clive, and their attorney. The psychological clearance letter would state that all parties had been counseled prior to the start of our arrangement; that we all understood our roles, responsibilities, and expectations; and, more importantly, that surrogacy would not impact our lives negatively.

We needed to buy medical insurance for Victoria, and we knew that there might be a long waiting period before she would be covered for pregnancy, so we decided to start looking into medical insurance first. We contacted an insurance agent whom I found on the Internet. My first question to him was, had he worked with people who had used his services to find medical insurance for surrogate mothers? He assured me that he had. I gave him all the information he requested, and I told him clearly that the pregnancy was a surrogate pregnancy and that we wanted to make sure all medical expenses for our surrogate mother were covered.

A couple of days later, the insurance agent contacted me with information about three different policies, each with a different price tag. He sent the information packet for each policy to both Victoria and I to review the details, and I contacted each insurance company to double-check his work. Would a pregnancy as a result of surrogacy be covered? I found that I had to ask the question in a certain way so that the agents on the telephone could understand my question. I explained to them that I was not the one who was getting pregnant; our surrogate mother was, and the policy was for our surrogate mother. They all basically said that they would not cover the surrogate mother getting pregnant, but once she was pregnant they would cover all medical expenses, subject to co-payments and deductibles. Fabulous! Apart from the cost of each policy the main difference was the waiting periods. I spoke to Victoria at length about each policy, and jointly we decided to use the policy with no waiting period. Before we signed on the dotted line, I asked the insurance agent to state in writing that the expenses would be covered. Once we received the letter, Victoria completed the forms and sent them in to the insurance company.

After Victoria's medical testing was completed, we arranged for her psychological evaluation. The evaluation consisted of a fifty-minute discussion with the psychologist, in which they discussed Victoria's role and responsibility and how she felt about bearing a child for someone else, and also about giving up the child after birth. Victoria always described herself as being an "oven," so that is what she told the psychologist. After the consultation she had to take a personality test, which consisted of about 500 questions.

While Victoria was taking the test, the psychologist called Craig and me for our evaluation. We spoke to her for about an hour, and we basically talked about our thoughts and feelings about the prospect of someone else carrying a child for us. I relayed to her that I am typically an impatient person by nature and that I would have to try, somehow, to curb my natural instinct to be demanding in this way. Victoria knew me better than I thought she did, because she also mentioned this to the psychologist in their discussion. I don't know what the result of their conversation was, but I was glad I discussed it with the psychologist. She explained that this would be a natural reaction, so I felt much better. She also explained that I might start to have feelings of jealousy, and that it would be a natural response to our situation. The question was how would I handle it? I was glad that the issue of jealousy was raised, because I had never thought about it before. I was so busy making arrangements that the thought never crossed my mind.

I had always got along very well with my brother Clive. We were great friends, in fact. One of the concerns I had about this arrangement was that something would happen that would destroy our friendship. I hoped desperately that this would not be the case.

The result of our discussion with the psychologist was that she thought that Victoria would be a perfect surrogate mother. At the conclusion of our telephone consultation, she said that she would be available for discussion if Victoria or I needed to talk further. Our psychologist sent a clearance letter to the fertility center, which basically stated that each party had been evaluated and there were no issues to speak of.

That evening I decided to ask Victoria how she knew that she could hand the baby over to Craig and me at birth. She said that because she'd had two children of her own, she knew exactly how she had felt and would feel after the birth. Immediately after the births of both of her own children, she described a short period of detachment. After a little while her maternal instinct would kick in and she would then bond with her baby. It was in this period of detachment that she knew that she would have no problem giving the child to us. I now understood why it was a requirement of the fertility center for the surrogate mother to have given birth to her own children.

As we started to go through this journey, I started to learn a lot about all sorts of things. I learned a little more about Victoria. I always thought she was a strong, stable, and level-headed person. Now that we were doing this, I started to feel in awe of her.

What a strange feeling this was. Here I was arranging everything for a pregnancy, and I wasn't the one who was pregnant! I was the "administrator" of this pregnancy. *Is this what the psychologist meant when she said that I would feel jealous?* Maybe; maybe not. I don't know.

The next step in the process was the legal side. Where would we find an attorney? We decided to tap into the resource we already had. The fertility center gave us the name of a law firm, so we made contact with them and spoke to one of their attorneys. The attorney we dealt with actually turned out to be very nice, and quite responsive to our questions. I guess I was expecting the same kind of treatment we received from our IVF doctor in New York. The attorney explained that after we paid the retainer fee they would be our resource—from the commencement of our journey to when the baby came home with us and our names were on the birth certificate—without any additional legal fees. In summary, their services were to (a) prepare the contracts and make any necessary changes, (b) prepare the final legal clearances for the fertility center, (c) prepare the legal pleadings to declare my husband and me the legal parents of the baby, (d) coordinate with the hospital, (e) write a hospital information letter with the legal judgment in advance of the birth, and then (f) assist us if we had any issues that came up at the hospital at the time of the birth, or during the birth certificate process. We asked the attorney to send us her firm's information.

We received the retainer agreement from the law firm. We decided that we would wait for all the medical test results to come back before we retained the attorney. It looked like the whole journey was going to be quite expensive, so we didn't want to pay out money when we didn't have to. We all agreed that this was a good idea.

As expected, the medical test results were favorable for us to start our journey to having our own child. Victoria would be a perfect surrogate mother! I was really excited. We were on our way, hopefully, to becoming pregnant!

Now that we were given the go-ahead medically, the next thing we needed to do was get our contracts drawn up. We paid the retainer fee and our attorney sent us a standard contract. We reviewed it carefully, line by line. One of the great things about going through this legal process was that our attorney was available via e-mail. If we had questions we sent her an e-mail, and shortly afterward we received a reply. This was good, because sometimes when we called the office she was either on the telephone, in a meeting, or in court. If we needed to speak with her we would send her an e-mail and make an appointment, and then she would either call us or we would call her at the appointed time. It was a very good arrangement.

The standard contract was a very detailed document that covered everything from who each party was and who would have custody of the child upon birth, to the surrogate mother not consuming products or medication that would harm the child.

The contract also itemized the payments we had agreed to make, such as medical insurance, maternity clothing allowance, gas, and co-payments to the doctor. We would pay for all medications and for a house cleaner, as soon as Victoria felt she needed one. We did not want her to be out-of-pocket for anything related to the pregnancy. She was already giving us so much. The least we could do was make sure that this was not a financial burden to her in any way.

We had spoken to Victoria at length about each part of the contract, so it was no surprise that when the contract was sent to Victoria's attorney for review there were no changes that needed to be made. Her attorney sent a letter to our attorney stating that he had reviewed the contract on her behalf and there were no changes. Victoria and Clive signed the contract and sent it to our attorney. Craig and I signed our copy of the contract and sent it back to our attorney. We now had a fully executed contract in place, so our attorney sent a legal clearance letter to the fertility center. The clearance letter basically stated that we had a contract in place and that all parties understood and agreed to it.

We decided to purchase life insurance for Victoria, because we felt that if anything happened to her during this elective process we wanted to make sure that at least her family was covered financially.

5

We Are Ready to Get Pregnant

How odd to think of "we." *We* now included my husband, me, and my surrogate mother, Victoria!

The medical tests were completed, and the psychological and legal clearances had been sent to the fertility center. We were now ready for Victoria to become pregnant.

The fertility center we chose in California coordinated my treatment with my reproductive endocrinologist (RE) in New York. Even though we didn't like our RE in New York, we felt that because I had actually produced eggs with the protocol I was given, we should to stay with her. We were happy that the management of our case would be handled by Dr. Batzofin's office.

What a great feeling it was to go to the RE in New York and not have to be concerned about getting two minutes of her valuable time to explain things to us. I just needed her to do the sonograms and testing. If we needed to have anything explained to us, I could contact Dr Batzofin's office. I did not need her to do anything else. The two fertility centers were so different—like chalk and cheese, night and day. Our new fertility center seemed to have all the time in the world for us. Not surprisingly, we felt quite hopeful and a lot less worried.

I was amazed at how easy it was to coordinate our requirements across country—for example, Victoria's medication. She took the prescription to the pharmacy and left it with them. Eventually, someone from the pharmacy contacted me for payment information, and then the medication was shipped overnight to Victoria.

For my medication it was just as simple. The fertility center in Pasadena would fax instructions to my RE in New York, and when I went in for my next scheduled visit I would be handed my prescriptions. I would fill them as usual at the pharmacy I had used before for my IVF treatments. Fortunately for me, the only payment I had to make for my medication was my co-payment. I was still covered under the insurance I used for my IVF cycles. We had to pay for all of Victoria's medical testing, sonograms, and medications. It really was very expensive already, and we'd only just started!

Victoria and I were each provided with our own calendar from our fertility center in Pasadena. It told us exactly what medications we should take and how much, and when we needed to go in for a sonogram or blood work. This was really helpful, as it kept me on track if I had any doubt as to what medication I needed to take, and when. I was tied to this calendar, and I was constantly double-checking to make sure that I was doing the right thing at the right time. I couldn't bear the thought of the cycle not working or being cancelled because I had made a mistake and not done something when I was supposed to.

It would take three cycles to prepare us both for the transfer. The object was to synchronize our cycles. I was amazed at such a thing. I didn't know that you could synchronize cycles. The first cycle started when Victoria started her period and was instructed to take the birth control pill every day.

The second cycle started when my period started eleven days later and as directed, I took my birth control pill daily. On day 21 of Victoria's cycle she was instructed to take Lupron and also continue taking the birth control pill until her next period started. Lupron is used to desensitize the ovaries so that the cycle can be controlled. I was used to taking shots from my previous cycles of IVF but I was worried about Victoria taking her first shot. I wondered if she would find it painful and decide that she did not want to go ahead with everything, but she did not complain at all. In fact, I had to ask her if she had any feelings that were different than usual. She said that she had a headache, but she didn't complain at all about taking the shot. I started to have a headache with my medications, too, but I am not sure if my headache was caused by the medication or by my constant worrying. I guess it must have been the worrying, because I don't remember having a headache during my previous cycles of IVF.

I continued taking my birth control pills until day 20, when I was instructed to start injecting myself in the thigh with Lupron daily. I was now taking my birth control pills *and* Lupron. On the twenty-fourth day of my cycle, I was instructed to stop taking the birth control pill. Every night I continued to inject myself with Lupron while I waited for my period to start.

My period finally came, and this was the start of the third cycle. I called my doctor to let her know that my period had started, and I arranged to go in for blood work to check my hormone levels and a sonogram to check my ovaries. During this time Victoria started taking Estradiol every couple of days, and she also had blood work done to check her hormone levels and sonograms to check whether optimal endometrial development had occurred. Estradiol was administered to prepare Victoria's uterine lining for implantation of the transferred embryos.

Part III
Egg Retrieval and Transfer

6

First Trimester

Week One: I went to my doctor's office for blood work and a sonogram. The results were faxed over to the fertility center in California so that they could review the results and make adjustments to my medication, if necessary. No adjustments were needed.

On day 9 of my cycle I was instructed to start taking GonalF and Pergonal. GonalF and Pergonal were given to stimulate my ovaries to increase the number of mature eggs that I would hopefully produce. My husband would give me the shots in the evening. By this time he was an expert at mixing and administering all the medications. He would clean the site with an alcohol swab, mix the sterile solution with GonalF and Pergonal, suck them up into the syringe and then inject me in the bottom. He became very good at it, because none of the solution was ever wasted.

I would wonder how I could go through all this pain and heartache and *still* not be pregnant. Whenever it was time to take the shot I would bury my head in my pillow so that my husband would not see the pain on my face. I would also pray that this time we would be successful.

I developed numbness in both of my thighs. I first noticed it when I would lie on my side, and then suddenly my thigh would start to tingle and be really uncomfortable. I ran my fingers up and down the area and realized that the numbness was in the areas where I had injected myself in the thigh with Lupron. On my next visit to my RE in New York, I asked her about it. She explained that I had probably hit a nerve when I gave myself the nightly Lupron shots. She also explained that the nerves would eventually knit themselves back together and all should be well. *All this pain, discomfort, upset, and worry. How much more pain and suffering would we have to endure before we became pregnant?*

I was excited about going to California to prepare for the retrieval of my eggs and meet the doctors and nurses at our chosen fertility center for the first time. I would be traveling with lots of syringes and vials of medication, so I was given a note from the doctor in California that explained the reason for all the syringes I was carrying—just in case my bag was searched at the airport. Armed with medication, syringes, and my growing follicles, I boarded the plane to California. Sitting on the plane and looking out of the window, I tried to visualize the multiple follicles growing in my ovaries and prayed they would survive and be very healthy and strong.

I arrived safely, and I was happy to see that Victoria looked well. Since Craig would be arriving a few days later, Victoria would give me my nightly shots of Pergonal and GonalF. She was very nervous at first, but she soon got over it.

Week Two: I went to see Dr. Batzofin and his staff for the first time, and I was really nervous. I hoped that he would not be dismissive, as I had found our previous doctor to be. I took a deep breath and waited in the waiting room until my name was called. I gingerly walked into the examination room, sat down, and waited for him to come in. Although my impression of the doctor was very good during my telephone consultation, it was a relief when I finally met him. When he came in I found him to be very warm and welcoming. Even though I could tell he was busy, he answered all my questions and did not rush me at all. He encouraged me to ask as many questions as I wanted to. This was a great relief. During my examination, he performed a sonogram and said that I had three follicles in my left ovary and three in my right ovary. I asked him if there might be a possibility of there being more, and he said that it was not likely. This was okay, because six eggs were retrieved from my previous IVF cycle, using the same protocol. All I needed was one good one.

The next day Victoria had her appointment with Dr. Batzofin. She had a sonogram, and her uterine lining measured 14.7 mm. I understood this to be a good measurement for pregnancy, and I was very happy and excited. The doctor printed off the sonogram picture, and in the middle of it he'd typed "Let's get pregnant!!" I thought that this was very funny and very encouraging, and I was happy that we had chosen this fertility center.

The next day I had my follow-up sonogram. Dr. Batzofin said that the eggs were not quite mature enough and scheduled me for another appointment a couple of days later.

I went in for my follow-up sonogram, and this time my eggs were mature. We would definitely be doing the retrieval on the scheduled date. At last, our retrieval date was confirmed. I started to feel very nervous and excited at the same time. *Surely it would work this time.* I really hoped it would. I took the shot to induce ovulation, as directed, and we waited anxiously for our appointment to arrive two days later. Craig arrived that night, and he was bright and cheery as usual. I was a bag of nerves.

How would we pass the time until our retrieval appointment? I could not sleep. Not sleeping was becoming a regular habit of mine. Lying awake at night—wishing, praying, and hoping—was adding to the time we had to wait. Getting pregnant was proving to be more stressful than I had ever imagined. I don't know how, but somehow or other we made it through.

Week Three: Our retrieval day finally arrived. I was tired when we got up, but I was living on nervous energy and managed to function quite well. We were all excited and raring to go. I kept my fingers crossed all the way to the fertility center. We were greeted with cheery smiles from the nurses, as usual, which put us at ease somewhat.

I had decided to have a general anesthetic for the procedure. I did not want to move or feel any discomfort during the process. While I was being prepared, Craig was given a little container and told to go to another room and donate his sperm into the container provided. Later he would describe the room as being a storage room, and the entertainment provided was 1970s *Penthouse* magazines. He also said there were women waiting outside to have their blood drawn from a nurse in another room. This did not stop him, as he was very keen and ready to go. When he was finished, he came out of the room and smiled at all the women, while raising his container as if he were toasting everyone. "Morning, ladies," he said happily. Craig was not embarrassed at all.

I was lying on a bed in the treatment room, waiting for my procedure to start, when Craig came into my room with a beaming smile on his face. He had just seen his sperm under a microscope and he said they were waving at him. He was very proud!

During the egg retrieval process, a vaginal probe was inserted into my vagina and a needle guide was inserted along the probe. Using ultrasound, the needle was directed into the ovary to aspirate an egg from each follicle. Once all follicles had been aspirated from one ovary, the needle was moved to the other ovary to remove the eggs. Each follicle was examined by the embryologist to see if it contained an egg. The eggs were then incubated, and, using the intracytoplasmic sperm injection (ICSI) procedure, each egg was injected with a single sperm to hopefully achieve fertilization.

Shortly after I woke up from the procedure we were told that six eggs were retrieved, and I was happy because six was the expected number. I rested for a short time and was given discharge instructions, which included not lifting anything heavy for twenty-four hours. I was assured that someone would call me the next day to let me know how many eggs had fertilized and how many embryos we would have. I envisioned that they would all fertilize, as they had done with my previous IVF procedures. If there were six embryos, the plan was to transfer three to Victoria's uterus and then cryopreserve (freeze) the other three in the fertility center's storage facility. Embryo cryopreservation, or embryo freezing, is a method used to preserve embryos by cooling and storing them at low temperatures. They can then be thawed at a future date and transferred to the uterus, providing additional opportunity for achieving conception. Because our previous IVF treatments had not been successful, I was convinced that we would be unsuccessful the first time and we could use the three frozen embryos for a second try.

We felt very optimistic the next morning, before we received the call from the fertility center with results of our fertilization. One egg had fertilized, and two eggs did not survive due to poor quality. My optimism was short lived. I wondered what had happened to the two eggs that did not survive. I went and had a look at my calendar, which I had followed religiously to keep me on track of what to do and when. *Hadn't I taken my medication when I was supposed to? Hadn't I had the sonograms when I was supposed to? How come they did not survive?* The nurse said there could be a number of reasons, and we would need to talk to the embryologist and the doctor to get the details.

We still had three eggs left, which hopefully would develop into three healthy embryos ready for transfer. I understood this of course but my heart wouldn't accept it. I started to feel really upset again, because I had visions of this cycle being a total bust. Even though I suspected that we would not succeed on the first try, I was still disappointed and hurt. I tried to sound optimistic to everyone, but disappointment was written all over my face. Again that night, I did not sleep at all.

The next morning I could stand it no more. At 8:30 AM I called the fertility center to find out if they could give me more information about our retrieval. Another embryo had fertilized. This was very good news. I asked about the remaining two eggs. There was still no progress on those two. As we were going to have our transfer appointment the next day, they said that they would let us know the progress of the last two eggs when we arrived for our appointment. Every thought and feeling I had about the remaining two eggs were negative. I had another sleepless night. Even though I had disappointments in the past, I was still not used to this feeling of defeat and helplessness. I knew that we didn't have the final results yet, but I still felt deflated.

Craig drove Victoria and me to the fertility center for our transfer. It was pouring with rain, and there was a lot of traffic on the road. I felt that I wasn't the only one in a panic, and that was a comfort in a way. We all felt stressed, and we asked Victoria if she knew of another route to get to Pasadena. We took a supposed short cut to avoid the heavy traffic. We avoided the traffic, but after a while I had lost my sense of direction and prayed that we would not end up in Los Angeles! I feared that if we didn't get to the fertility center on time they might cancel our appointment. The likelihood of this happening was probably remote, but I felt the stress nonetheless, because I hate to be late for anything.

Finally, we arrived. We were greeted with the warm, welcoming smiles of the nurses. There was no problem at all. What a relief!

We learned that the last two eggs had fragmented. Fragmentation occurs when the cells of an embryo split off into smaller fragments. A certain amount of fragmentation is considered normal and is not harmful, but an excessive amount is indicative of lower-quality embryos. So from six eggs, two embryos had fertilized and four did not survive. I felt the backs of my eyes prickling with tears. *It is not going to work again*, I kept repeating to myself. The procedures had failed in the past, and the procedure was going to fail again. Somehow I had to gear myself up for the transfer. I tried to be optimistic by saying to myself that we only needed one embryo to implant. Our two embryos were graded "A," which was excellent quality. This was encouraging news, but I still felt pessimistic.

Everyone at the fertility center was cheerful and smiling. How could I be the only one who felt miserable? I wished I had someone to talk to, or something to read that would tell me that my upset feelings and thoughts were valid and real. I was the odd one out. I managed a little smirk. I felt such a fraud. Victoria was hopeful and smiling, so I felt a little more encouraged and my smirk developed into a little smile, but I'm sure she could see right through it.

In order to prepare for the transfer, Victoria had to drink a lot of water. This was so that during the ultrasound her uterus could be visualized clearly. When everyone was ready to start the procedure, a speculum was inserted into her vagina and her cervix was cleaned. Victoria was told to cough as Dr. Batzofin placed a catheter through her cervix and into the lower segment of her uterus. The embryologist had already transferred our two embryos to a finer plastic catheter and this was placed through the outer transfer catheter and placed near the top of her uterus. The ultrasound was used to visualize the lining of the uterus and guide Dr. Batzofin in the placement of the catheter. Once the placement was correct, the embryos were expelled from the catheter and inserted into her uterus.

I was in the room during this monumental occasion when our two embryos were transferred. Craig waited in the waiting room. Victoria was excited and eager. It felt good to be a part of the procedure. Craig and I would be going home in a couple of days and I really felt that I wanted to have the memory of the embryos being transferred to Victoria fresh in my mind. The transfer went very well, and the staff was pleased. Victoria rested for a short while in the treatment room and was given discharge instructions. These instructions explained that Victoria should be restful during the first twenty-four hours and engage in only limited activity during the second twenty-four hours.

On the way home Victoria lay down on the back seat, and we all prayed for success. When we got back to Victoria's house I started to clean and scrub everything that was in my path. I worked really hard so that Victoria would not have to do any work, but I guess I did it mainly for myself so that I could keep my mind off the day's events. Victoria started her nightly progesterone shots to help the implantation process. She did not complain at the sight or size of the needle. The needles were quite large compared to some of the needles I had used. I remembered from my IVF procedures that I developed lumps in the areas where the shot was given. I wondered whether Victoria would develop lumps on her bottom, too.

7

We Are Pregnant!

Week Four: Craig and I went back to New Jersey. We had left our two precious embryos behind, being well looked after and taken care of in Victoria's uterus. They would hopefully grow to be our children. I felt like we were carrying the weight of our future on our shoulders. *If we were unsuccessful, how would I go through each day?* I did not dare to answer this question for fear of jinxing everything.

It was Monday, and I was back at work. No one had any idea what we had done the previous week. When I started to feel anxious, I would close my office door and sit quietly and pray.

I called Victoria to ask her if she was going to test to see if she was pregnant. She emphatically said no. I was disappointed because I wanted her to test. I wanted to know. I needed to know. Suppose the first test was negative? I would have asked her to go out and buy a different test, as I had done after each IVF treatment I had. From experience this could have gone on for days, so in the end I was glad that she didn't want to test. I would have driven Victoria crazy, and I did not want to do that. Victoria is very calm by nature, and I found that her personality forced me to try to be calm as well.

Instead of driving Victoria crazy, I drove my dear friend Fiona crazy. Fiona had struggled with infertility in the past and managed to become pregnant while taking Clomid, which helped her to ovulate. Whenever I was feeling down, she knew exactly what to say and how to make me feel better. She validated my feelings and made me feel worthy. With her help, I was able to feel a lot less anxious about everything.

With my past IVF cycles, I had a blood test to check my hormone levels seven days after the transfer and then a pregnancy test fourteen days after the transfer. This is known as the two-week wait period. Victoria would be going to the fertility center for a blood test to check her hormone levels eight days after our transfer. There was no point in working myself up into a frenzy before the official pregnancy test. While we waited I daydreamed about babies. I found an IVF Web site where people were in their two-week wait period, and I read what they had to say. It wasn't the same, though. I was still looking for someone who was going through the same process as I was, so that I could share my anxieties with them.

Victoria went to the fertility center to have her hormone levels checked eight days after the transfer. It was a normal day for me and nothing major was going to happen until day 14. On day 14 we would know one way or the other—if we were pregnant, or not.

The telephone rang at about 5:20 PM, and it was one of the nurses from the fertility center. After pleasantries were exchanged she asked me if I was sitting down. I wondered why she would be asking me this, because we still had another five days to go before the pregnancy test.

"Victoria is pregnant!" she said. I sat down. More than likely I fell onto the chair. I could hardly speak. "She is?" I managed to stammer. The nurse went on to explain that Victoria would be going in for another blood test in a few more days, and she probably said a lot of other things, too, but I didn't hear a word. *Pregnant* was all I heard. I was dumbfounded. How could it have worked on the first try? What a wonderful surprise…Happy New Year!

Shortly after my conversation with the nurse, the telephone rang again. This time it was Victoria. She was calling to tell me that she was pregnant. Y I P P E E! All I kept saying was that I could not believe it, and this fantastic news just would not sink in. Victoria was very proud that she was pregnant, and she had an air of success about her.

The blood test showed that the level of the pregnancy hormone hCG was 31.54. Apparently if this number was greater than ten, it meant that she was pregnant. Well, it was definitely greater than ten! When Craig came home I told him the exciting news. We were ecstatic, and we went out for dinner to celebrate. It felt like a dream. It felt unreal. It *was* unreal, because it wasn't me. I was not the one who was pregnant.

I could not wait for the next blood test results. I was so excited and on tenterhooks. I would smile for no reason at all. I found myself on the Internet, researching the pregnancy hormone levels to try to predict what the next result would be. Apparently, if the number doubled every other day then the fetus was developing as it should. Victoria went in for her second blood test, and I called the nurse to get the results. The hCG level was 396! Wow! The number more than doubled every other day. I wondered if there could be more than one fetus. I asked the nurse, and she said that we should wait until we did the sonogram. More waiting. I couldn't stand it.

I got in touch with our attorney. I wanted to make sure that we could stay ahead of anything we needed to do from a legal standpoint. I wanted to have a smooth legal process with no catastrophes. Our attorney said that we could begin the legal process of the finalization of parental rights about halfway through the pregnancy. She would need to know which hospital we would be using for the delivery, so that she could send the judgment to the administrator of the hospital and instruct them to put Craig's and my name on the birth certificate. At this time we didn't know which hospital we would be using. I would have to make sure that the OB/GYN and hospital were covered by both Craig's and my insurance, as well as by Victoria's insurance. When the baby was born, he or she would be put on Craig's insurance (mine would be used as a secondary insurance if we needed it), and we did not want to have to switch hospitals because of an insurance glitch.

Victoria went in for another blood test a few days later. The hCG level was 8911. Again the number had more than doubled every other day. *How can there not be more than one?* I asked again if there could be more than one. The nurse said that she was very pleased with Victoria's results, but we should wait for the sonogram to reveal the actual number of fetuses.

We scheduled the sonogram for February 6, 2001, at 11 AM. I immediately booked my flight to California. I would not miss this for the world!

Week Five: I wondered how we would make it through each day. I was so excited that I couldn't stand it. I was sure there were twins. I couldn't wait to go to California to find out.

Craig and I created two tapes of our voices so that Victoria could play them to our baby. I wondered if other people had done this. We wanted our baby to hear our voices and get used to us as soon as possible. We told our baby how much we really wanted him. I told him that my tummy was broken and that I couldn't carry him inside my tummy, so Victoria was going to keep him nice and warm for us until he was born. We read nursery rhymes and sang lullabies, and recorded them. We found that we had so much to tell him. We told him about our days at work and where we were going to put his swing set in our garden. I asked Victoria if she could play these tapes to our baby as often as she could, and she said that she would.

Was it possible that our baby could reject us if he or she did not recognize our voices? Was this a strange thought to have? Our baby would not reject us, because he or she would know exactly who we were. With Victoria playing our tapes and me going to visit as often as I could, he should know exactly who I was when he was born.

Part IV
Our Pregnancy

8

Twins!

Week Six: I arrived at my brother's house in California at midnight. I could not get there quickly enough. I willed the appointment for the sonogram to come as quickly as possible. I enjoyed the weekend activities with Clive and Victoria's children, and that passed the time nicely. On Monday I worked remotely. What a wonderful invention the laptop was! My work was quite flexible. As long as I could communicate with whomever I needed to when I was supposed to, then everything was fine. I was glad that I had something to concentrate on. Monday night arrived—the night before our appointment. Again I could not sleep. I kept tossing and turning. I wondered how many fetuses there were. I had a really strong feeling that there were two. My mind wandered from strolling through the park with a baby in the stroller, to no pregnancy at all.

Victoria had been throwing up a lot. I had no idea that she would be so sick. In a way I was very glad, because if she was throwing up that meant that she must still be pregnant. I also felt sad, because it must have been very uncomfortable for her. She started to eat crackers to make her feel a little better. It didn't help, though.

I looked at a week-by-week pregnancy calendar, and at this stage the heart should be developed and the eyes and ears were beginning to form. I wondered if we would be able to see any of this on the sonogram. Hopefully, our baby was developing normally.

Week Seven: We went to the fertility center for our confirmation of pregnancy sonogram. Victoria had her blood taken for her hormone levels to be checked. We then had to wait in the waiting room for the sonogram. Victoria's name was called and we both went into the treatment room. After what seemed like an eternity, Dr. Batzofin came in. He did the sonogram and it was almost immediate that we saw TWO SACS!!! I could not believe it. Not only that, we could see their hearts beating, too! It was fantastic. How lucky I felt. After all the nights of worrying about having only two embryos, both of them had implanted.

What were the chances of this happening? To be honest I didn't really care. I just cared about Victoria being pregnant—and with twins, no less.

Dr. Batzofin said that the first twin measured six weeks and two days, and the second measured six weeks. Because the second sac was a little smaller, he wanted to see its development at the next sonogram. I started to worry immediately, and I knew that I would not sleep a wink until the next sonogram.

After reviewing Victoria's blood test results, the doctor said that she could change the frequency of the progesterone shot from every day to every other day. The blood test results were perfect.

Victoria had progressed from crackers to bread. She had thrown up quite a few times by this point, and I started to feel really guilty. *Surely being sick was a good thing, wasn't it?* But when I heard her throwing up, it didn't sound like a good thing at all.

I flew home a couple of days later, and I felt every emotion in the book. I was happy that we were pregnant and sad that Victoria was so sick. I was sad that I had to leave and I was anxious for the second twin—and for the first twin, for that matter.

Week Eight: Victoria had an appointment that was scheduled for 8:30 AM her time, 11:30 AM our time. I felt sick, and I couldn't eat or drink. I was so worried about the smaller twin. I had read everything on the Internet about the vanishing twin syndrome, and of course it made me feel even worse. The vanishing twin syndrome is when one of the fetuses in a twin pregnancy spontaneously aborts. This usually happens during the first trimester, and the fetal tissue is absorbed by the other twin, the placenta, or the carrier, thus giving the appearance that the twin "vanished".

At 11:45 AM our time we could stand it no more. Craig called me and said that we should call Clive on his cell phone. We called Clive and he told us that he was taking care of his children in the waiting room while Victoria was being seen by the doctor. They'd only just arrived, and Dr. Batzofin had just arrived also. Nervously we hung up the phone and waited for it to ring. At 12:30 PM Victoria called and said the second twin was still there and should be there to stay. What fantastic news! I was so relieved. It was Valentine's Day, so we had two things to celebrate.

Victoria told us that the doctor videotaped the sonogram for us, and she would be sending the recording to us in the overnight mail. I didn't know that you could video tape a sonogram, but I was really excited that we would be able to see our fetuses.

When we received the video recording we watched it over and over again. It was great to be able to see some of what was happening. They were beautiful. We even saw and heard their hearts beating. This made the pregnancy seem a little more real to us.

Now that the pregnancy was real, we started to think about names. This was another daunting task, but I felt sure that if we had two girls, their middle names would be Victoria.

Week Nine: Craig and I celebrated nine weeks of pregnancy. We felt that this was an important milestone, and it should be honored. We went into New York City and had a lovely dinner at a very nice restaurant. When we got home we watched the video recording again to see our babies' hearts beating.

At this point we had told only a few people. We really didn't want to announce our pregnancy to everyone because we had a fear that something awful might happen. I remembered our IVF failures and how awful it was to tell people that the procedures were not successful. We had got so far, and I did not want to jinx our luck.

I was worried every day. I was constantly thinking about how things were going. Not being in California with Victoria was really proving to be quite difficult. I had this overwhelming urge to be near Victoria. *Was it normal to feel this way? What would I do if I were there...follow her around?* Of course not, but I had this overwhelming feeling of wanting to be in Victoria's presence and share some of her pregnancy aura.

I was always the big sister to Clive and Victoria, but now I felt like the young child. In a lot of ways I felt completely powerless. Why was this? Victoria was pregnant, and I was not. I wanted everything to go right so that she didn't have to worry. I did not want to upset her. I did not want to be a pain in the neck. After awhile I felt like I was walking on eggshells, even when I was not in her presence. I didn't want to cause upset and make her have any regrets about carrying our babies. I wondered whether this was the jealousy feeling that the psychologist described in our consultation. Part of it probably was a bit of jealousy, because I would have loved to have the feelings of pregnancy. The other part was anxiety, because I was worried about everything.

I didn't call Victoria as much as I could have. I could have called her many times a day, but I didn't want to be a pain. How I controlled the urge I just don't know, but I did. I still spoke to my brother Clive almost every other day, and this was normal for us. So on the days that I wanted to call Victoria, I would talk to my brother instead and ask him about how she was feeling, and this sufficed. I thought that calling Victoria once a week was reasonable, although I had been talking to her more often when she had her appointments. It worked out to be more like three or four times a week, depending on what was going on. On some occasions when I had felt like calling her and I controlled the urge to do so, Victoria had actually called me. Maybe she sensed my anxiety; I don't know.

During this time, Craig and I sat down to watch a program on the Discovery Health Channel called "Eggs for Sale," about egg donation. It was an hour-long program, and we had unfortunately missed the first half of it. There was a woman on it who was talking about Lupron and her fertility injections, and I was glad because at last I could actually hear and see someone else talk about their experiences with IVF. Egg retrieval day came and she was in her doctor's office getting ready for the procedure, and I remember thinking, *Wouldn't it be funny if the doctor was Dr. Batzofin?* A couple of seconds later the doctor started talking. *No, it can't be*, I thought. The doctor then came back into full view on the television screen, and there was Dr. Batzofin! I could not believe it. Of all the fertility centers in the entire country to choose for the program, it was the one with my doctor in it. Unbelievable! What a good choice I had made.

The program showed the egg retrieval process, which was good for me to see because I had been anesthetized for all of my retrievals. The eggs were fertilized, and after much discussion the couple decided that they would not mind having twins, so they agreed to transfer three embryos. A few weeks later they found out they were pregnant with twins. Amazing!

9

When Do I Tell People?

I had been having many tortuous thoughts about being dishonest with some of my really good friends. I had literally avoided any verbal contact with some of them for a very long time. Yes, we'd communicated via e-mail, but there was so much that I did not have to say in an e-mail. Thank goodness, because I couldn't cope with the sound of betrayal in my voice.

The main reason I didn't want to tell many people about what we were doing was because of our previous IVF failures. We were devastated when we found out that we were not pregnant, and we had so many people to tell that it hadn't worked. If this surrogacy failed, for whatever reason, I did not want to have to tell anyone. It just would have been too much.

Of course I could have telephoned some of my friends and talked to them, but I would have felt such a fraud for not telling them what was going on. I lived and breathed having a baby, and it was on the tip of my tongue. What kind of conversation would I have if I were concentrating on not telling them what was really going on?

My old school friends in the United Kingdom and I were planning to get together on June 22 to celebrate our fortieth birthdays. I had said that I would go, but I knew that if there was something I needed to be present for at that time I would be off to California without hesitation. I knew they would understand, but I just couldn't help feeling that I was being dishonest.

It was the same with friends who were close by. I hadn't told them a thing. When asked whether we were going to continue the IVF treatments, I just said that we were going to try again in the summer.

Brenda, a friend of mine, is a therapist, and I swear she knew my secret. She asked me at the beginning of February if I wanted to talk about our struggles with infertility and our IVF treatments, and I said no and some other rubbish about having a break. But I felt so dishonest because I had told a big lie. I was glad that she did not ask me any more about it. The worst part was she said that she was my friend and wanted the best for us, and if I wanted to talk about it to call her. UGH! This made me feel even worse.

10

Worry, Worry, Worry

Week Ten: I don't think I had worried so much about anything before. I felt that I was in constant turmoil. I prayed daily that everything would be okay. I prayed for no deformities, no congenital defects, and no problems. Being the administrator of our pregnancy made me feel really mechanical and logical. I had arranged contracts and payments, scheduled appointments, and so forth, and I just didn't feel like a mother-to-be at all.

I was amazed by the video of the sonogram showing the embryos, the sac sizes, and the heartbeats. I had seen the sonogram, received the results of the blood test, and had it confirmed by Dr. Batzofin and the nurses, but it was still unbelievable to me. I still couldn't believe that Victoria was pregnant.

Victoria went in for her appointment the next day. I spoke to her at 3 PM my time. Everything was fine. Dr. Batzofin was very pleased with her progress. He said depending on the results of the blood test, her hormone levels might reveal that she could come off all medications completely. He also said that this visit would be her last visit at the fertility center because she was doing so well. Victoria had already made an appointment with her GP to get a referral to an OB/GYN. Victoria called and told us that she would not have to take any more shots. I was really glad about that, because I knew that her bottom was getting very lumpy.

Victoria said she had another video recording of the sonogram for us and she would overnight it to us so that we would get it as soon as possible. I couldn't wait.

In last week's conversation with Victoria, I found out that she doesn't enjoy being pregnant at all and absolutely does not want to have any more children of her own. I knew that she didn't want any more children, but I was so shocked that she didn't enjoy being pregnant! I thought it was just the morning sickness she didn't like, but it's the whole thing! That just made me even more in awe of her. She was doing this for us from her heart!

We received another video cassette of the sonogram today. It was so great to see our babies. I couldn't wait to hold them.

We were getting close to the time when prenatal tests could be done. I had been doing a lot of research on amniocentesis. Amniocentesis is where a small sample of the amniotic fluid surrounding the fetus is removed and examined. It is used to diagnose chromosomal and genetic birth defects such as Down Syndrome and it is usually performed during week fifteen to week eighteen of pregnancy. It also reveals the sex of the babies. I had been very worried about this test, because there was a 1 percent chance of a miscarriage. Also I had read that they might be able to test one twin but not the other, because of the position of the second twin. At this time we decided that we were going to have the test done, no matter what. We needed to know before the birth if there was going to be a problem, so that we could decide what to do and prepare for it.

Because I felt so distant from everything, I followed a pregnancy calendar weekly to help me see the development of a fetus. The pictures I saw were not of my fetus, but at least it gave me an idea of where we should be in terms of development. At ten weeks of pregnancy our babies should be moving around, and the elbows, wrists, knees, shoulders, hands, feet, fingers, and toes should be formed.

Week Eleven: Poor old Victoria was still very sick. It seemed to be getting worse. I thought it would improve because she had stopped taking the progesterone, but no joy there. She said that she stayed in the car when her son was playing soccer on Saturday because she felt so ill. She did manage to watch some of his game, though. It seemed to me that the actual throwing up had increased, because before this she was just feeling nauseous most of the time. I felt guilty because I couldn't help but feel that this was a good sign for me. It told me that she was still pregnant and her hormones were still raging. I felt terrible, on the other hand, because she was suffering so much.

At this stage I found that I was desperate for information. I couldn't find anything anywhere. Every piece of information was directed at the pregnant woman—which makes perfect sense, of course—but what about me, the intended mother, and how I felt? Was all the worrying I was doing normal? What about my mental confusion? I felt so alone. I could talk to Craig, to a point, but he is very matter-of-fact about things, and also male. I would have liked to have read a book about the intended parents' feelings that would then validate some of my feelings, such as the overwhelming urges I had about wanting to be in Victoria's presence all the time. *Was I crazy to feel this way? How would I overcome it? Was this feeling normal?* I couldn't find the answers to my questions. What about the worry of something horrible happening to them all? These were real feelings I had, but I didn't have a point of reference.

The psychologist who gave us our psychological evaluation said that it was going to be difficult, because I was going to feel jealous of Victoria being pregnant and me not. Well, I think that I was too worried to be jealous. I was the administrator of this pregnancy—a much needed function—but I did feel very removed from everything, and this was perhaps why I wanted to be around Victoria all the time.

My other worry was phoning Victoria too much. Ideally, I wanted to have news every day, but this of course was totally unrealistic. I didn't want to come over as being too needy or too pushy or too anything. I am typically an impatient person, but somewhere along the way I learned how to be patient because Victoria is so calm. The funny thing was, Victoria had been calling a few times a week, which was great. Perhaps she sensed that I was trying my hardest not to be a complete pain in the neck.

I was also worried about something happening that would destroy the relationship I had with my brother. This was another reason why I was so anxious about everything. I hated this feeling, because I felt so inadequate. I had to accept that this was what was going on at this time. Hopefully, after our babies were born I would regain my senses, and be back to normal again.

We needed to start thinking about what we were going to need for our babies. I wanted to go to Babies R Us, but Craig said that it was too soon, and he wanted to wait. I really wanted to go. Maybe I was just being impatient again. Okay, I decided to wait. I started to collect articles about twins and lists of what we would need when they came home. The mound of articles was piling up. We were going to need a lot of stuff.

Victoria phoned and asked me for information such as the date of my last period, date of birth, and so forth. She needed this information for the appointment she had scheduled with her general practitioner. She said also that she was going to take the first available appointment with the obstetrician-gynecologist (OB/GYN) that she was referred to. She was having the same feelings that she had with her daughter and her son, that is, sickness and feelings of preterm labor. Preterm labor is when you start having regular contractions that cause the cervix to start to open or thin out (called dilation and effacement) before thirty-seven weeks of pregnancy is reached. It was imperative that she be seen right away. As if I needed anything else to worry about! I was now worried about this. I was going to be upset if I couldn't make the appointment, but the priority was for Victoria to be seen by a specialist as soon as possible.

I found that I was talking to myself all the time. I had to. I didn't really have anyone else to talk to who really understood what I was going through. I would tell myself things like *take each day as it comes, one step at a time,* and so on.

Here I was again, wanting to tell everyone what was going on—but I couldn't. At first I thought I would wait until the end of the first trimester, which was the twelve-week mark. But then I thought that maybe we should wait until the results of the amniocentesis. That was going to be around the middle of April, which also meant that we would not get the results until the end of April. I should have been used to having to wait for everything, but I still wasn't.

I was in the elevator at work one morning when a red-headed Australian woman got in. She was very friendly and started talking about my padded coat. "It looks very warm," she said. "Oh yes, it's like walking in a quilt," I said. "What is it made of?" she asked. "It's Downs," I said. Suddenly, I was mortified. I meant to say it was filled with down feathers, and I corrected my mistake. She didn't notice, of course, but I certainly did. Amniocentesis was constantly on my mind.

I telephoned Victoria at about 2:30 PM after the appointment with the doctor. I could stand it no more. She had just arrived home. I hoped she didn't think that I was too pushy, but I needed to know how things went at the appointment. She had been to her general practitioner (GP) and got her referral to see an OB/GYN, which fortunately was just across the hall from her GP. I thought that she would have been referred to a perinatologist, who is a specialist in high-risk pregnancies, but that was not how it worked with the insurance plan that we had purchased for her. All specialist treatment had to be coordinated through the OB/GYN, who apparently had treated high-risk patients before, according to Victoria's GP. The OB/GYN's business card read "OB/GYN and Infertility." I got a bit nervous about the doctor specializing in multiple things—like our doctor in New York, whom we ended up not having much faith in at all. Anyway, the fact was that that was the insurance plan we had, and that was how it worked. I really hoped this doctor was on the ball.

Victoria told me about a couple of books to read. In one of them there was a very informative section about problems that can occur during pregnancies with twins, such as preeclampsia (high blood pressure and the presence of protein in the urine), preterm labor, diabetes, and so forth. I decided that I would transfer the warning signs mentioned in the book to my notebook, and every time I talked to Victoria I would check the symptoms on my list. If there was anything unusual, I would ask her to call her doctor. I was sure that Victoria would be doing this anyway, but I just wanted to make sure.

Victoria explained a little more about how she was feeling. She said that she felt like she did when she was pregnant with both of her own children at the time they found that she had preterm labor. Even though the scare was real, she was still able to carry both of her children to term. I asked her to describe the feelings to me. She said it felt like contractions, when her uterus would tighten up. She said she felt good on one occasion, and she did the laundry. After a while the contractions started, so she sat down and rested, and then felt much better. Resting seemed to do the trick.

Victoria made an appointment with the OB/GYN. Thankfully, they could fit her in. She had a list of questions for him and she also planned to tell him about the contractions. One of the things she hoped to get from the OB/GYN was a timetable of events. I wanted to be present at as many appointments as I could, but I needed to know in advance so that I could coordinate the time off from work and make travel plans.

If this doctor suspected that Victoria needed specialized treatment right from the start, then he could actually refer her to a specialist now. I hoped he would refer her, and I hoped that she could be seen quickly by the specialist.

Victoria felt nervous about going to the doctor's office. When I asked her why, she said that she thought they might look down on her because the babies she was carrying were not hers. Fortunately, both doctors' offices were happy for her. She was congratulated by her regular general practitioner and also by a nurse in the OB/GYN office.

I felt quite sad because I had wanted to attend this appointment with her, but everything seemed to be moving along very quickly. Again I was waiting anxiously to see what the new doctor said. Victoria called and said that she spent thirty or forty minutes with him. That seemed to be a long time to spend with a doctor, but he was very thorough in his evaluation. He told her that he had dealt with high-risk pregnancies and surrogate pregnancies before. I was happy to hear that. She explained all the relationships to him: Victoria was carrying her husband's sister's and brother in law's babies. She went on to tell him that she felt she was having contractions, and he told her that she would know when she was overdoing it—so basically, no more laundry, cleaning, and so forth. She needed to have a lot of rest. He also told her that she must eat more regularly, and that the food should contain lots of protein and iron.

Regarding the schedule of appointments, he said that he wanted to see her in four weeks, at which time he would take more blood, do another sonogram, and talk in more detail about the amniocentesis and other tests that could be done.

He would then refer us to a genetic counselor, if necessary. I would definitely be able to attend the next appointment, which I was very happy about.

The doctor did a sonogram on Victoria's belly, and he was able to see two babies—both moving normally and their hearts beating normally. He said that if he had not been told there were twins he might not have picked it up at this stage, because of the way they were positioned. He said he had to really search for number two.

I was in research mode again, and I wanted to learn as much as I could about amniocentesis. Apparently, this was the most accurate test at this stage. As far as I understood, it was 99 percent accurate. The alpha-fetoprotein (AFP) screening test was another test that we could do at this time. It would measure the protein level in Victoria's blood. An abnormal result would mean that we could have an amniocentesis to find out more details. However, the numbers could be off for twin pregnancies, so the AFP was not accurate for multiples.

The rate of Down Syndrome is higher the older you are. At this stage I was thirty-nine, and Victoria was thirty-five. There was a 1 percent risk of a miscarriage with amniocentesis. What a hard decision to make! On one hand, I wanted to do the test to find out if everything was okay. On the other hand, I couldn't bear the thought of Victoria having a miscarriage because of it.

I found this week of the pregnancy to be particularly difficult. I had been reading everything in sight and worrying about everything I had read, to the point of getting really upset about it. Why I did this I will never know, but I felt that I needed to know as much as possible about all of our options.

I spoke to Victoria about doing the amniocentesis, and she said she would be happy to do it. Basically, there was no point in doing any of the other tests. The results of those would probably be inaccurate and/or inconclusive, because there were twins. I felt much better after talking to her. We really did want to know the results of the test that would show the most results, so we decided that we would go ahead with the amniocentesis.

The schedule so far was that the next doctor's appointment was on April 6 to do blood work, a sonogram, and to talk about the amniocentesis and other tests. The doctor would then give us a referral to the genetic counselor for two weeks later. Craig and I would fly to California for the appointment with the genetic counselor and for the amniocentesis, and two weeks after that we should get the results of the test. After that I was going to go to California every month until the appointments were more frequent, and then I would take it from there.

Week Twelve: I was so happy to have reached this mammoth milestone. We had another cause to celebrate. We told some of our closest friends and family that we were expecting twins, and it was truly wonderful. Everyone was really happy for us. They were just amazed that surrogacy could be done medically, and that someone would actually carry someone else's child. At last I could talk about our journey. It was really good to be able to unburden some of the load I was carrying. However, I was still looking to share experiences with someone who had actually gone through or was going through the surrogacy process.

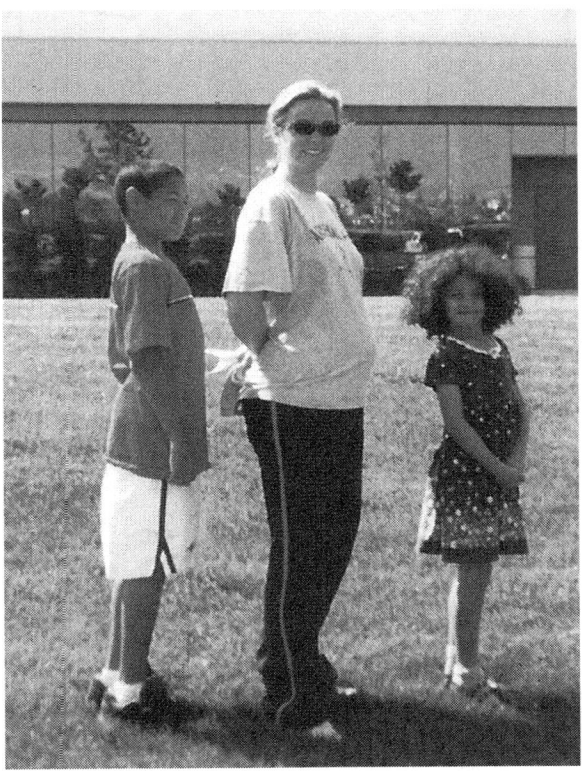

Victoria, three months pregnant, with her children, Marcus and Chloe.

Poor old Victoria was still very sick. I spoke to Clive, and he said that she was having more good moments than bad ones. He also said that she felt about five months pregnant. She was eating a lot and resting, also. These babies were going to be born with very nice weights indeed. She had been reading some books and had learned a lot about eating well and eating often, and resting.

I was still looking for information from an intended parent's point of view. I had searched high and low for a book written from my point of view, and I couldn't find one anywhere. Even on the Internet there was nothing. There were lots of books about adoption, but this absolutely was not the same thing. It would be really nice to find something I could read that would validate my feelings as being normal, and would also tell me the kind of feelings that I might expect to have. Even if I didn't go through any of them, it would be nice to see someone on my side.

I had read a couple of books that I found to be very interesting but they were more process-oriented rather than feelings-oriented. After I read them, I still felt that there was something missing. Was it a big secret? How come there wasn't anything? What books were other intended parents reading? I realized that I would have to write the book that I was looking for.

11

Second Trimester

Week Thirteen: I decided that each step was going to be very hard and I was going to worry about everything, so I might as well just accept that fact.

I couldn't wait for our babies to arrive. Craig and I kept on talking about the things we were going to do with them. At the weekend we talked about getting a swing set for them, and we discussed where in the garden we were going to put it. We were also going to get them a sandbox. We would need some shade in our garden, so we would have to plant some trees.

Craig suggested that we go to Babies R Us. I was ecstatic. I had wanted to go for such a long time. I was excited that he'd made the suggestion and that he really wanted to go. I had suggested this a month ago, and he said it was too early. Anyway, we walked in, and I suddenly felt like I was going to be swallowed up as the walls started to close in on me. I must have been having some sort of panic attack. I felt overwhelmed with stress and strain. The store was massive. I started to sweat and feel faint, so I went outside and took some deep breaths. After a short while I felt a little better. I took some more deep breaths and decided to go back into the store.

We started off in the stroller section, and there were so many different brands. *Twins,* I remembered in time, so that narrowed the selection down. We weren't going to buy anything, just look around. Where do we start? Which stroller, car seat, high chair, crib, mattress, clothes, bottles, diapers, and so forth? It was much different from buying something for yourself, because then you don't buy everything at once. And because I am a research freak, I can research that one item for myself and not be overwhelmed by it. But this! This was something completely different. Where would we start? The other added complexity was California. We were going to need things there, as well. I knew that we would need car seats, clothes, bottles, diapers, and so forth there, so we decided that we would buy those items the next time I went to California.

We looked around the whole shop, and I felt like I was being swallowed up with each step. I was walking around in a daze. Craig asked a very nice assistant to explain the car seats to us. It was a good thing that Craig was there, because he seemed to be taking in what the sales assistant was saying. My head was spinning. We finally left, and I felt relieved. Craig had taken in a lot of information, so I decided that he could fill me in on everything later when we got home. After I got home, I felt much better. I wondered whether I was going to have a panic attack every time I went shopping for baby items. I sincerely hoped not.

Week Fourteen: We received an e-mail from our lawyer. She said that she would be petitioning the court between the second and the third trimester, so that by the six-month mark we would have a judgment from the court. She would also prepare the legal paperwork and circulate it to Craig and me, Victoria, and Clive's and Victoria's attorney for signature. Once a judgment was obtained, which usually took only a few weeks, she would obtain certified copies and mail them to us and the hospital, with instructions to place Craig's and my name on the birth certificate. She would also coordinate with the hospital, so that they would be aware of the situation and then make sure that everything ran smoothly. This was good to hear. It really looked like we were not going to run into any legal issues. Our names would be on the birth certificate and the hospital would already be informed. That was exactly what we wanted.

Week Fifteen: I flew out to join Victoria at the next appointment with her OB/GYN. It was a roller coaster day for me—again. We went to the OB/GYN, who was a very nice man who seemed to have a lot of time for us. He gave us lots of information, and we were able to ask lots of questions. He asked whether we were going to do the amniocentesis, and I said yes. There was a flash across his face, which looked doubtful. The long and the short of it was that without him actually saying no, he was implying that he didn't think it was a good idea to do the amniocentesis test. The most obvious reason was that Victoria was already suffering with preterm labor, so her odds were much closer to falling into the 1 percent miscarriage rate. He said that the odds might be one percent, but if it happened to us it would be 100 percent.

The doctor went on to say that they didn't usually test both twins. I had read that the only time they didn't test both twins was if the second twin was in an unreachable position. I told him this, and he then said that they fill the first one with blue dye to make sure they don't test the same baby twice. I had also read that. I asked him to give us a recommendation, and he basically said he would leave the decision to us. He also said that if it was our second or third child he would have no hesitation in recommending the amniocentesis test.

I spoke to Craig on the phone, and basically I decided this was too great a decision for me to make on my own, without all the information from the genetic counselor. Craig would be arriving in a couple of days, so all three of us would go to the appointment with the genetic counselor. If we decided to do the amniocentesis and ended up losing two perfectly healthy babies I would be devastated, and I was sure Victoria would be, too. Not only that, but depending on the nature of the miscarriage, Victoria could have problems—or worse still, she might end up losing her uterus.

I spoke to Craig on the telephone the next day, and we decided not to do the amniocentesis. It was too great a risk to take. I couldn't imagine that Victoria would want to go through all this and endure the morning sickness all over again. We were going to have a very detailed sonogram. If they found something that was not right on the sonogram and they recommended amniocentesis, only then would we go through with it. That seemed to be the best solution.

Week Sixteen: I noticed that Victoria was rubbing her belly a lot. I had seen her do this before, but it seemed more pronounced on one particular afternoon. She stood up at about 4:30 PM and said she was going to bed, to get some rest. I felt encouraged, because resting was good for her. A short while later, her son came down from her bedroom and said that he would have to stay with a neighbor that night, because his mother might have to go to the hospital. I immediately ran up to her bedroom, and she said that she felt like she was in labor. I started to panic. She said that she wanted to wait for another hour to see how things went. No way! I immediately arranged for her children to stay with a neighbor and I drove Victoria to the hospital.

I found a wheelchair for her, wheeled her into the reception area, and informed the receptionist that Victoria was going into labor and was only sixteen weeks pregnant. Even though there were quite a few patients waiting, we did not have to wait long at all. Soon after all the insurance details were given, Victoria's name was called. We went into one of the examination rooms to be seen by a nurse and doctor. Victoria told them what her symptoms were, and they recommended a sonogram. We then went to the sonogram area, where they did a very detailed sonogram. They looked at the head circumference, kidney, diaphragm, stomach, and lungs of each baby.

We also saw the sex of our babies. We were going to have boys! Two of them! It was really exciting to see. We could clearly see that the first twin was a boy. The second one was a little more difficult, but eventually we saw that he was a boy. We were going to have to start with the names all over again, because we hadn't got around to choosing any boys' names yet. I was really glad that they were healthy and doing well. Victoria's uterus measured sixteen weeks. Twin A measured seventeen weeks and Twin B measured sixteen weeks and one day. They were both a bit bigger than the average, which apparently was really amazing for twins.

Victoria was told that she would have to go on strict bed rest—no going up and down the stairs. She could go to the bathroom, but that was about it. At the doctor's instructions we scheduled a follow-up appointment with Victoria's OB/GYN for the next day. Victoria went to bed when we got home. I wondered how she was going to stay off her feet for the next five months. I hoped that there was a pill that she could take, otherwise my guilt levels would go off the charts.

I was glad that I was there. I went shopping with Victoria's children and I loaded up two shopping carts with lots of food and fun stuff for the kids to eat. I was happy that I could do a lot of practical things so that she didn't have to worry. I started to worry about what was going to happen when I was not there. It had been a very stressful day. Craig would be arriving that night, and I couldn't wait to see him.

At this stage we really needed to find a facility that had a level three neonatal intensive care unit (NICU). The hospital that our OB/GYN was affiliated with went up to level two. This was a big concern for me, because if our boys came early and needed level three treatment, would they get to the level three unit in time? I made a note to ask the doctor if he was affiliated with a level three hospital.

We went to the OB/GYN, and he prescribed Brethine for Victoria to take every four hours. This medication relaxes the uterus to prevent contractions, but doesn't affect the babies at all, apparently. He explained that she would probably have to take this medication for the rest of the pregnancy. I could tell that Victoria was relieved to know that there was a preventive step that she could take. I asked the doctor if the hospital he was affiliated with had a level three neonatal intensive care unit, and he said no. He assured us that if there were any complications that required level three attention, the hospital was more than well equipped with procedures and equipment to transport very sick infants to the nearest level three facility. Hopefully, we would not have to put this to the test.

We decided to tell my old school friends in the UK at this time. I sent them a really long e-mail that summarized what we had been going through trying to get pregnant, and that Victoria was now pregnant with our twins. I apologized for not getting in touch with them sooner. I received e-mails from them expressing their sorrow for what we had gone through and congratulating us on our pregnancy. One e-mail I found to be particularly touching was from my friend Su, whom I've known since I was twelve. Here is what it said.

Dear Sandra,

I downloaded e-mail yesterday and there were twenty-three messages. I responded to Christine and another friend Sarah straight away, but felt that I really needed a bit of time to digest yours more fully. I've read and re-read your email so many times today and it just blows my mind.

I don't know what to say first. Mainly I just feel so absolutely delighted for you both I can't tell you. My daughter Milly is the hardest work at times, but without doubt the best thing that has ever happened to me.

I am completely in awe of Clive and Victoria. To have a baby (babies!!!) for someone is just so incredible I just can't get my head around it. That's love.

I can completely understand that you haven't wanted to talk about it all. Sometimes when times are tough it's much easier to retreat.

There's so much I want to say and to know—I'm all of a jumble. Twins!!!!! Wow. I can only try and imagine what you've been going through. Wow—you'll have two boys.

I wish more than anything that you weren't so far away. I often feel like that, but even more so now.

I totally understand about the fortieth bash. Of course you can't make it. It was so lovely to hear from you. I was getting very worried that we wouldn't talk anymore.

Love and kisses,

Su

Receiving these kinds of e-mails and good wishes from our friends and family made us feel really great. Everyone was full of encouragement and they had only positive things to say. Everything was going really well.

12

Meeting with the Genetic Counselor

Week Seventeen: We went to see the genetic counselor. We did the sonogram, but it was a bit of an anticlimax because I thought that this sonogram was going to be more detailed than the one at the ER the previous week. The doctor confirmed two boys. She took head measurements and thigh measurements (apparently some defects can be identified by this measurement), looked at their stomachs, and saw four chambers in their hearts—thank goodness. And that was that. Everything was in the normal range, and she couldn't tell us anything else. The previous week the doctor in the emergency room really went to town. She measured everything. One thing the emergency room doctor said was that we would be surprised by the equipment used in other places. I thought she was talking about the doctor's office, not the genetic counselor's office! You could hardly make out what was on the screen, but we were able to see our boys kicking each other. Craig was happy to see this.

Victoria had her blood drawn for an AFP (alpha-fetoprotein) test. The AFP test measures a protein that is released from the baby into the carrier's blood stream. The test is used to estimate the likelihood of birth defects such as spina bifida and Down Syndrome. This screening test does not diagnose a specific condition, but it does indicate the probability that the baby is at risk for certain defects. The problem I found was that unless you were forever the optimist—and not a worrier like me—these tests were designed to scare you to death. The AFP test produces a lot of false positives. For example, the test could say that there was a probability of having a child with a defect, but then you would have a healthy baby. That would be fantastic, of course, but while you were waiting for the birth you would be really worrying.

The genetic counselor advised us to do an amniocentesis because the eggs were produced when I was thirty-nine years old. This was getting to be very stressful. We couldn't do an amniocentesis, because Victoria had preterm labor symptoms that were now under control, thankfully. If we were to do the amniocentesis and it caused a miscarriage, I didn't know what I would do. No, we decided to wait until we saw our OB/GYN again. If something was revealed on the scan and the doctor advised us to do an amniocentesis, then we would do it. But as long as the decision was ours, no amniocentesis would be done.

In the meantime we confirmed that our boys were going to be covered under my husband Craig's medical insurance. We contacted Craig's benefits office and were told that we had thirty days after the birth to send in the paperwork that added our boys to our policy. I was glad that the administration part of all this was going well.

Victoria had started to eat again—thankfully—and had not been sick for two days. She was trying to figure out which pill was making her sick—the iron pill, the folic acid, or the calcium pill. I didn't think it was any of the pills. She was carrying two babies, and they were both sending her hormones raging.

Week Eighteen: The doctor's office called to give me the results of the AFP test. Using my statistics, the nurse said that there was a 1 in 59 chance of having a baby with a defect. The probability was calculated using the due date of the babies and my race and my age. I wasn't sure which due date was used, because the due date had changed a couple of times. First we were given the beginning of October as a date, and then we were given dates based on the size of our fetuses. So using one of these due dates, my age (thirty-nine), and my race (Black), they came up with the probability of 1 in 59. Using Victoria's age (thirty-five) and her race (Caucasian), there was a 1 in 192 chance of having a baby with a defect. I asked the nurse why there were two calculations done, and she informed me that they did the calculation using Victoria's age for their records. The fact was, though, that the eggs were mine, so the probability of a defect was 1 in 59. I telephoned Craig immediately and told him the results. We decided that I would go to Victoria's next appointment with the genetic counselor, which was scheduled for a week later.

As each phase passed, I felt that I couldn't possibly be more worried than I was during the previous phase. There was worry at every step, and I was distraught again. With the AFP test result we would now be eligible for an amniocentesis, and it would probably be recommended by the doctors. I didn't want to have the amniocentesis, but now that we had the results, the counselor was recommending that we have it. This was all incredibly confusing and upsetting, because the results represented a statistical chance, and I did not know if the results referred to one baby or both. I confirmed the appointment to discuss the results with the genetic counselor. Victoria and I would attend the appointment and learn the details together. I would then discuss the details with Craig, and we would all make a decision.

With a heavy heart I booked a flight to go to California for the following week. Victoria had scheduled an appointment with the OB/GYN for the day before the appointment with the genetic counselor, so I would be able to attend that appointment as well. I found that I wasn't able to function very well. I had that awful feeling of not wanting to get out of bed again. I had read everything there was to read about the AFP test, and I could not get any encouragement from anything. *How was I going to make it to the next week?*

Week Nineteen: Each day seemed to drag on, until finally the day came for me to go to California. *Why was everyone smiling when I was so miserable?* The genetic counselor was going to confirm that we should do the amniocentesis and I was going to be devastated.

We went to the appointment with Victoria's OB/GYN. He was so helpful and really did seem to have all the time in the world for us. When we went in for our appointment he said that the genetic counselor was on the phone and asked whether we were going to tomorrow's appointment. Absolutely I said. After he hung up the telephone he asked us what we were going to do about the amniocentesis test. I told him that only if they found something out of the ordinary on the sonogram would we do an amniocentesis. He was pleased. It appeared that he didn't want to tell us what to do but my interpretation of his comments was that he did not want us to do the amniocentesis. He asked whether the genetic counselor's office had put any pressure on us to have an amniocentesis. This was a very interesting question I thought because I did feel that they had wanted us to do the amniocentesis. I told him this and we had all decided that we would only have the test if any blood tests or sonograms had unfavorable results. I felt much better that our doctor was happy with our decision.

The night before the appointment with the genetic counselor I could not sleep a wink. I watched each second, minute, and hour go by until it was time to get up. The morning of the appointment I felt really worn down with worry and stress. My shoulders were the tightest they had ever been and I could barely turn my head.

Our appointment with the genetic counselor was at 10:15 AM, and we got there about 9:30. They were running late, of course, and we were eventually seen at about 11:00. We went into the counselor's office, and she informed us that she was on the phone with the testing facility because she didn't like the results. *How can I say this without losing control again?* I immediately went into a state of panic, and I felt myself trying to get every ounce of me to not lose control. I was so upset that I just couldn't keep it inside any longer. I felt like I was going to explode. I started to cry and cry. Victoria tried to comfort me, but my mind kept on repeating what the counselor had just said—she didn't like the results. I could not control myself as I kept on crying.

Finally the counselor finished her conversation with the lab, and then she told us that the calculation was wrong. The results that were given to us prior to our appointment were based on the wrong due dates. I was crying so much that I couldn't speak. *Was this a good thing or a bad thing?* I wanted to ask, but I was too choked up to communicate anything other than how upset I felt. She apologized and said that maybe she should have had the conversation with the testing facility while we were not in the office. Duh!! Really! Some people can be so stupid. She knew I flew out specifically for this appointment, so to anyone else this might have suggested worry and concern. Some people just don't think! Anyway, she finally gave us the results. She said the due dates were off by ten days—which way I don't know, because I was too upset to ask. With the new date change, my chances for a defect came down to 1 in 360. The cutoff line for the amniocentesis test was anything below 1 in 190, so I didn't even come close. They also did a calculation for Victoria, and her results changed to 1 in 1759. Because of this new result we did not qualify for another sonogram or the amniocentesis. We would have to wait for Victoria's next scheduled sonogram, which was in the middle of May.

The counselor also said that the original probability she had for me was 1 in 78, and for Victoria it was 1 in 250. These were totally different from the numbers the doctor's office gave us, where mine was 1 in 59 and Victoria's was 1 in 192.

I really didn't know what to say! I was so relieved to see that my numbers had improved dramatically, but after leaving the counselor's office and mulling it over for a few days, I was really cross thinking about how upset I had been for the last week! I did understand how the problem arose, though. We were given a due date of October 4 by the fertility doctor. We had another date that was based on Victoria's last period. Then we had another date based on the size of the babies (which were ahead of schedule). We should have had the test through the genetic counselor's office, not the doctor's office. But according to the insurance, we had to do it through the doctor's office, and because of that everything was a fiasco.

The genetic counselor was incredibly insensitive, and she really should have recalculated the numbers without us being in the office while she was on the phone. She should have called us in when she had all the information. We had already waited an hour and a half. What difference would another fifteen minutes have made? I felt drained and exhausted, and I couldn't wait to go home.

13

I Am Going to Be a Mommy!

Week Twenty: This was a huge milestone, and Craig and I celebrated it accordingly with a lovely dinner.

Here I was again, wanting to be near Victoria. I had only just come home from my visit! I felt really powerless. I had always been the one Victoria and Clive looked up to, and now I was looking up to them. I was in complete awe of the fact that someone would actually carry a child for someone else. For this I would be eternally grateful. I also felt a shift in "power." I was not in control of this situation, and therefore I felt helpless and vulnerable. I was not used to this feeling, and I didn't like it at all. The reason I wanted to be near Victoria so much was because I wanted to feel some of the feelings she had. I knew that this was crazy, of course, but I really wanted to be in her glow of pregnancy.

Every time the telephone rang, I hoped that it would be Victoria. I hadn't told Victoria and Clive about these feelings because I didn't want them to think that I was losing it or something. I always felt so happy after I had spoken to her. Even if there was no change or nothing much to say, I still felt happy.

Week Twenty-One: Our attorney sent us an e-mail to let us know that she was going to petition the court so that we would have the birth certificates issued in our names. This was very good news. The administrative side of this was going really well. I had no complaints at all.

Victoria called after her sonogram appointment. She had a different doctor do the sonogram this time, and this new doctor said that everything was perfect. She measured their heads, arms, legs, abdomen, hearts, stomachs, diaphragms—everything, really, and all was well. I was so relieved. All the measurements were the same, too. Both babies and Victoria's uterus all measured twenty-one weeks!

I had been looking at a pregnancy calendar, and according to this calendar my boys should weigh about a pound each. I had read that if they were to be born now, there would be a strong chance of their surviving. I called and asked the

OB/GYN about this, and he said that the chances of their survival were much better around week twenty-six. Obviously, the longer they were in Victoria's womb the better off they would be. This was still a real concern for me because of Victoria's history with pre-term labor. I prayed every day that everything would go well with my boys and Victoria.

Week Twenty-Two: Victoria called me to let me know that the boys were doing fine and had started kicking. I was so happy to hear from her. Again I wished I was there. After I hung up the telephone, I felt really low. I wanted to feel my boys kicking inside of *my* tummy, but, sadly, this was a feeling that I would never, ever have. I wondered how it would feel to be carrying a life inside of you. How great, powerful, and strong one would feel. I looked at the pictures of the sonograms Victoria had sent to us and tried to imagine how it would feel. I tried really hard, but I just could not imagine the feeling.

Week Twenty-Three: I just got an e-mail from Victoria! It made me really happy.

Hi Sandra,

Just to let you know everything is going fine. The movements of the boys are getting stronger each day. I do seem to be slowing down quite a bit and also having to eat smaller meals. Each day I get bigger, so that means the boys are growing. Speak to you soon, Victoria.

I was so amazed by Victoria—I really was. I knew that I was idolizing her, but I couldn't help it. The fact that she had gone through so much for us—I just could not get over it.

Week Twenty-Four: Now that we were getting closer to week twenty-six, I started to feel more certain that I would be a mother. I had heard of babies surviving with very low birth weights, so I felt that ours could survive also. Their weights had always been a little more than what was stated in the pregnancy calendar at each stage, so deep down I felt comfortable that if anything happened, they would be okay.

Week Twenty-Five: I received an e-mail from our lawyer, who told us that the court had signed our pre-birth orders. Our names were going to go on the birth certificates as soon as our boys were born! Yippee! What a great day this was!

Everything was going perfectly. The major hurdle of getting the paperwork signed by the court had been done, and in plenty of time for the birth.

I flew out to California and went to the doctor's office with Victoria. We had another new doctor do the sonogram. We had already received a glowing report from one of Victoria's neighbors who had seen this particular doctor before, so we felt good about seeing her for the first time.

While we were waiting in the waiting room for our appointment, Victoria felt Baby B move. I put my fingers on the area and pushed down a little, but I didn't feel a thing. I kept my fingers in the same position on Victoria's belly, and then I felt a very light movement under my fingers. I was so excited! It really was real. I wanted to jump up and down and tell everyone that we were going to have a baby. Again I thought what a great feeling it would be to feel the movement of life in your body. While feeling the baby kick, I wondered again what it would feel like to have a baby move around in my own belly.

Finally Victoria's name was called, and we went into the treatment room for a sonogram. The doctor said that my boys were developing beautifully. They were exactly where they should be, developmentally. I was engrossed in trying to fathom out what was happening on the screen and trying to take in everything the doctor was saying, when suddenly the doctor asked Victoria if she was all right. I looked over at Victoria, and she was as red as a tomato. *What happened?* We had to stop the sonogram. The doctor got cold, wet cloths and put them on Victoria's head and around her neck, and then told her to turn onto her side. Apparently it is very common for pregnant women with twins to become very dizzy and feel faint if they are lying flat. Victoria sat up and had a cup of cold water. She felt fine after that.

After a while the doctor started doing the sonogram again. She was examining Baby B and said that his arm was in front of his face. I tried really hard, but I couldn't even see his face. I could see a hand, though, but it seemed to be just there by itself. The doctor pointed to where the face was, and then all of a sudden I could see that he had his right hand across his face. A tear came to my eye. I had waited so long to see this. What a sight to behold! A comfortable feeling came over me again, and I just felt that everything would be all right with my boys.

Week Twenty-Six: I was so glad that we had got to this milestone. If our babies were born at this time, there would be a strong possibility of their survival. I could now tell the people I hadn't already told. I couldn't wait to go home and tell the neighbors! Craig and I had decided that now was the time to buy the cribs, bedding, and other stuff, and we would do this when I went home. I wondered whether I would have another panic attack in Babies R Us.

I really was going to be a mommy!!!!

What a wonderful phase this was to be going through. When I got home, I arranged to go over to my neighbor Hannah for a cup of coffee and a chat. I told her that I just got back from California, and she said that I must really have a lot of work to do out there, because I was going there quite a lot. I explained to her that I wasn't exactly telling the whole truth about working out there. I then went on and said that I went there to visit my brother and sister-in-law, because Victoria was having our babies for us. Well, what can I say? She was absolutely bowled over with shock. I found it quite amusing, really, and very enjoyable. She kept on saying "What?" in a high-pitched voice. After she had got over the surprise, she asked many questions and was happy that I had someone who was willing to do this for me. Hannah was very happy for us all.

I went on to tell other neighbors and my colleagues at work. One of the surprising things I found was that once I had told people about our struggles with infertility, they would go on to tell me about their struggles, or they would tell me about people they knew who had struggled. I really didn't realize how difficult it was for people to have children. Fortunately for most of these people, they either went on to have their own children or adopted, or they accepted the fact that they would be childless and then moved on with their lives.

Week Twenty-Seven: I was absolutely distraught again. I received a call from Clive, who told me that Victoria had been rushed to hospital again with pre-term labor. That poor girl. She had gone through so much for us. *Please don't give birth now, Victoria,* I kept on repeating. I knew that I was happy to get to the twenty-six weeks point, but I really didn't want the survival theory to be put to the test. I frantically called all airlines to see what time the next flight was to California. I managed to get a flight for the next morning at 8 AM. Here I was again, counting the seconds, minutes, and hours to the time I had to get going to the airport.

I got to the airport with no problem—outwardly at least. Inwardly, I was a nervous wreck. As I sat there on the plane, I was so upset. No one knew how I felt or how powerless I felt. There I was in the air, and I was cut off from communicating with the people I needed to answer my questions. *Was Victoria all right? Were my precious, long-awaited boys all right?* Would I be able to keep calm for the next five hours? My throat was feeling really dry and constricted. I had a feeling that I was going to break down sitting there in the seat, up in the sky, five hours and three thousand miles away from where I needed to be. Fortunately I was sitting by the window again, and it was daytime. I stared out the window and got lost in the clouds. How many more times could I beg for everything to be okay?

As many times as I needed to, because here I was, getting ready to beg again. *Please, please let everything be okay with Victoria, and my two long-awaited boys.*

I arrived at the hospital at about 10:30 AM, and I was shocked to see the color of Victoria's skin. She was gray. All the color had drained from her skin. She was sucking on ice chips and feeling really sick. She had been given magnesium sulphate to stop the contractions, and unfortunately a side effect of this drug was nausea. She had severe nausea. Even though Victoria was really sick, the boys were still in their nice warm spot, growing and moving around healthily. What a weight off my mind! Craig was at home, probably pacing around and not knowing what to do with himself, so I called to tell him the good news. We both breathed a huge sigh of relief, but again I felt guilty that Victoria was so sick.

Victoria was released a couple of days later and ordered to be on strict bed rest. I wondered if she couldn't wait for this ordeal to be over. When we got home and Victoria was settled in, I went into crazy clean-up mode again and started scrubbing and cleaning everything, like I was a woman possessed. This was supposed to take my mind off the worries about early delivery, but of course it didn't. The good thing was that I was there to take care of things, and if we had to go to the hospital again I would be there, and not a whole day away.

Before Victoria was rushed to the hospital, she had made arrangements for us to visit the hospital's labor and delivery unit. I was very excited about going, because I could tell the people who were going to show us around that Victoria was carrying my boys. This always made me feel good. It also made me feel more involved. Fortunately, the tour of the hospital was a few days after Victoria was discharged, so she was well-rested for the visit. When we got to the hospital, I found a wheelchair for her so that she would not have to walk. This worked out well, because Victoria felt very comfortable in the wheelchair.

When we went on the tour, we discovered that there were four of us in the group. One woman was carrying quadruplets! We were not so unusual after all. We got a guided tour of the facilities by a very friendly nurse. The facilities were very nice, and Victoria felt comfortable about delivering at this hospital. They explained their transportation procedures to the level three hospital and even showed us one of the incubators a sick baby would travel in. We felt very comfortable when we left there.

When we got home I immediately sent an e-mail to our attorney advising her of the name and address of the hospital we had chosen for the delivery of our babies. She could now advise the administrator of the hospital of the legal judgment that had been granted which stated that both Craig and my name would go on the birth certificates.

14

Third Trimester

Week Twenty-Eight: Victoria was still very sick. It just broke my heart every time she got up to go to the bathroom. And still she did not complain. This could not be any fun for her, but not once did I hear her utter a word of regret about doing this for us. I felt so helpless and guilty that this was happening to her. When I talked to her about it, she said it was part of being pregnant. She really didn't seem to be bothered by it at all. Even though I knew that she had gone through this with her own pregnancies, it did not make it any better for me. She really was truly amazing.

Everything had calmed down by this point, and I was on my way home to New Jersey. As we got closer to the due date, I wondered when I should go back to California. I wanted to be there before the birth of the boys. The due date was October 4, 2001, so I thought that I would go out again toward the end of August.

Week Twenty-Nine: Craig and I went out and bought all sorts of things for the boys' room—two cribs, lots of blankets, diapers, clothes, bottles, and wipes. We spoke to many people who had children, and we made a list of the items they suggested we buy. It looked like we bought out the stores.

I never thought I had a creative bone in my body, but there I was painting stars and baby animals on the boys' walls. I painted the rhyme "Twinkle Twinkle Little Star" on one of the walls, too. I was so inspired and excited about everything. I wanted the world to know that our boys would be coming home soon.

Victoria was now scheduled to have two non-stress tests (NST) each week. Three monitors were put on her belly. Two were so that each baby's heartbeat could be heard. The third monitor was to monitor the contractions. They monitored the heartbeats to see if there were any signs of stress. So far, no stress had been detected.

Week Thirty: The feeling of wanting to be near Victoria was even greater than it had ever been. I wanted to rest my head on her tummy to see if I could hear or feel anything. There was no doubt in my mind that these babies would be born early, and I had this awful feeling that I was going to miss the birth. That would have just broken my heart. I was willing Victoria to carry my boys for a few more weeks. We needed their lungs to be strong, and I did not want them to spend any time in the neonatal intensive care unit.

I was constantly worrying about everything. *Would all this worrying ever stop?* I should accept the fact that I would be worrying about my boys for the rest of my life, because Victoria said that the real worry starts when the babies are born and you are worried about the baby getting a shot, getting a cold, and anything else related to your child.

I had been thinking about what I would tell my boys about their miraculous entry into this world. I had decided that once they knew what a tummy was I was going to explain to them that my tummy was broken, and that is why they were in Victoria's tummy. I looked forward to that day.

Week Thirty-One: Victoria went into hospital again with pre-term labor. I managed to book a flight and arrived in California the next day. I decided to stay there until my boys arrived. The doctors managed to calm the contractions and give her medications in pill form. She was released a few days later and was absolutely exhausted for a few days. The contractions really took it out of her. She started to feel a little brighter after a couple of days, and I was so glad to be there. My boys would be here very soon.

I was being a pseudo-mom by picking up and dropping off Victoria's kids all day, as well as going shopping and entertaining my five-year-old niece for most of the afternoon, so that Victoria could get a break. Things were going a lot better. Victoria was having contractions, but they seemed to be in the manageable range. The doctor called and told her that she must have lots of rest and lots of water, so I made sure she got what she needed. I did the cooking, cleaning, washing, entertaining, and everything else to keep the house going, so I was exhausted. *Heaven help me when I have my own brood!* Anyway, I was very happy to be there and to be able to do all those things for her. I was also very happy that I would be able to see the birth without having to dash across the country to get there. Victoria would be having a C-section, because the boys were not positioned for a vaginal birth. I was worried about this, because she had never had surgery before. My feelings went from anxiety and worry to guilt. *Will Victoria ever forgive me after the surgery?*

This pregnancy was really taking a toll on her body. She had been so sick. Oh, my goodness! I could still hear it, and she stopped hours ago. It was the most horrible sound, and it seemed to go on for a very long time. When she'd finished, she came out of the bathroom and said that she felt better. The poor girl was so used to it that it didn't even faze her any more.

While I was away Craig was on his own, and some neighbors had been rallying around and feeding him. One neighbor, Mia, cooked a huge pasta dish for him that lasted for days! That was really nice. He had also been invited over to a few neighbors on the weekend for a barbecue. He was having a great time.

Victoria told me that she put on fifty and sixty pounds, respectively, with her own two children, but she had put on only about thirty-five pounds with my two! At the last sonogram Twin A weighed four pounds and eleven ounces, and Twin B weighed four pounds and six ounces. These were fantastic weights for twins. It was amazing. She had an enormous belly, but when she had her back to you, you could not tell that she was pregnant!

Week Thirty-Two: I couldn't believe that we had made it this far. I was starting to feel really nervous. Something had happened to me, and I couldn't quite explain it except to say that I was feeling really anxious. Our boys could come any time now, and I didn't feel ready. I was prepared with cribs and blankets and diapers and so forth, but me, Sandra, I was not ready. I would have to be a grownup. *Was I ready to be a grownup? More importantly, would I be a good mother?* I hoped that I would be a good mother; I certainly would be trying my best. Why was I thinking about this now? I guess it was because I didn't have anything to organize, so those feelings crept up on me like a wave in the ocean.

Also, the possibility that Victoria would give birth soon was very likely. I jokingly told Victoria not to have the babies yet, because I wasn't ready. She thought it was the funniest thing. I guess no one is ever really ready. I had waited for the birth of my boys for such a long time, and now that the delivery day was nigh, I started to panic. *How was I going to manage two babies?* I started feeling really jumpy. I kept telling myself that I should be happy, and I *was* happy. I was just really nervous. *Was this how dads felt when they were waiting for the birth of their son or daughter? Maybe I should go out and buy myself a cigar and keep it in my top pocket, ready for the big day.*

Week Thirty-Three: I was in research frenzy again. I was trying to find out the cost of baby accessories—diapers, formula, anything related to a baby. I wanted to figure out where the best place to shop was. I knew that when I got home I would just buy the first thing I saw, but at that moment the research seemed to keep my mind on less important things.

The boys were really moving around a lot now. I had felt them kick a few times, which was always fantastic. How amazing it must be to feel a baby move around inside of you!

I started to wonder how Victoria would feel after the birth. Would she want to keep my boys? All along she had told me that the babies were Craig's and my babies, but I still wondered how she was going to feel. I had heard of hormones doing crazy things to pregnant women. Victoria kept assuring me that she was just an oven, and that was all. Whenever we were in a situation where people would ask how many months she was, in addition to answering their question, she would always tell the person that the babies were my babies, and not hers, which always made me feel good. I knew that I was feeling really insecure about this, but I really needed her to reassure me every now and again. We had a contract stating that the babies were Craig's and mine, but I really hoped that we would never have to refer to it. Deep down, I guess I knew that there wouldn't be any problems, but sometimes I couldn't help but wonder. I guess also that it was a mindset that she had put herself in. I understood again why a condition of surrogacy was that the surrogate mother must have already given birth and had her own children. Victoria knew how she was going to feel after the birth, because she had already gone through childbirth twice before.

Week Thirty-Four: Everything was going very well. We were going in for the non-stress test twice a week now. The NST monitors both babies' heartbeats and also monitors contractions. On Monday there were too many contractions, so they monitored Victoria for a much longer time than usual and decided to admit her. I thought that my boys would be born that night, but the doctors managed to stop the contractions again. Victoria was released the following day. Then on Friday, Victoria couldn't keep anything down, so she called the doctor and he told her to go to the hospital again. They monitored her again and the contractions were two minutes apart. The doctors managed to stop the contractions again, and this time Victoria did not have to stay overnight. This week we had three appointments—two non-stress tests and one doctor's appointment. Poor old Victoria. I tell you, she was such a trooper. Not one complaint came from her. It was amazing. The next Tuesday would be thirty-five weeks. If my boys were born now, I hoped that they would be all right. *They should be, shouldn't they?*

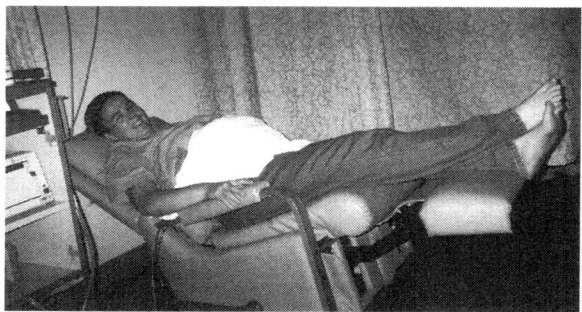

Victoria getting ready for another non-stress test.

Week Thirty-five: I was really looking forward to my hectic life with Craig and my boys.

My pregnancy calendar said that a baby should weigh about five and a half pounds at this stage. I knew that the weights quoted in the calendar were for singletons, but my boys were really big and healthy, and they could actually weigh five and half pounds each!

Craig had been at home every day, trying to keep himself busy until the birth. When he was not being fed by all the neighbors, he was doing a lot of gardening and also getting things ready for our boys' room. He managed to take everything in his stride. I, on the other hand, was still worrying about the birth and about getting to the hospital in time. I knew that our boys would be here very soon.

Part V
The Birth of Our Boys

15

Our Boys Finally Arrive!

Week Thirty-Six: What a day this was! It started off much the same as any other day, and then took a major turn. Victoria came over to me and said that she did not want to alarm me, but she thought that the babies were coming and we should go to the hospital. I rushed around the house trying to gather up things. I don't know what I was trying to do. All I needed were my shoes and handbag, but I was going around in circles. Finally, I took deep breaths to calm myself down. Victoria had already packed a bag for the hospital weeks before, so she was very organized and ready to go. She had also arranged for her children to stay with one of her neighbors, so all we had to do was get in the car and drive to the hospital.

I was going around in circles and trying to comprehend what Victoria had told me when the telephone rang. It was my friend Su, calling from the UK. I felt that my voice had risen a few decibels higher than normal, and I told her in a high-pitched voice that we were going to the hospital because Victoria felt that the boys were coming. Su was so happy and excited for us, and she wished us all well. I put the phone down, and I felt panic-stricken. I kept on telling myself that I was just not ready for the birth, but somehow I had to get Victoria to the hospital. I tried not to look panic-stricken, but I am not sure I succeeded. We got into the car and while reversing out of the driveway, I drove over the grass and some newly planted flowers. I had driven over this area of the grass many times, but never the flowers! I stopped to think about what I had just done and then I remembered that I had to take Victoria to the hospital. Hopefully the grass and the flowers would grow back.

While I was driving along the road, I heard myself saying all the actions I needed to perform in order to drive. "Mirror, signal, and maneuver," I said. I had to; I just couldn't help myself. Victoria must have thought I was nuts. It was as though I needed to hear someone tell me what to do, because I couldn't do it on my own.

We got to the hospital and I found a wheelchair for Victoria to sit in. I wheeled her straight over to the labor and delivery unit. The friendly nurses greeted us warmly, because by now we were regular visitors. After Victoria got into the bed, they immediately put monitors on her belly. There was a separate monitor for each baby's heartbeat, and another monitor to monitor the contractions. We waited for the doctor to decide whether he would deliver our babies straight away or delay the birth. We waited and waited for what seemed like forever. Two hours passed before we heard that he was in the hospital delivering another baby. I was glad that he was in the hospital, at least. By this time I must have walked miles up and down the corridor and in the little room where Victoria lay, waiting and resting. *Is this how would-be fathers felt?* I tried to watch the television. I tried to eat. I tried to read the newspaper, but nothing seemed to settle me. Finally, the doctor came in and looked at the printouts from the monitors. He told us that he was going to deliver our babies that day.

The moment I had been waiting for had finally arrived. I didn't know whether to laugh, cry, or worry. I remained silent because I was in shock. I could not move my body. I felt that I had something to say, but nothing would come out. Fortunately, Victoria was on the ball and spoke for me. She reminded everybody that I would be present in the delivery room, and therefore I would also need to get ready for the delivery. Finally, I managed to get out of my stupor. I gained the presence of mind to phone Craig and tell him that our boys were going to be delivered shortly, and that he should get here as soon as he could. He was very excited and said he couldn't wait for them to arrive. Craig reminded me to take some photographs. I had forgotten that I had my camera with me.

Victoria was wheeled off to the delivery room, and the nurses handed me some trousers, shoes, a hat, a mask, and a top—all made from blue paper. I was left in the room by myself as I struggled to put my paper outfit on without ripping it, because I was shaking so much. I sat on a chair and waited. It was very quiet in the room. I wondered if this would be the last time that I would hear quiet. I was shaking with excitement and relief. My boys would be here soon.

Suddenly, a nurse came bursting into the room and told me that they were ready for me. While we were going down the corridor to the operating room, she asked me if I had a camera. I had left the camera in the room! I ran back and got the camera and then ran to catch up with the nurse. We went bursting through two doors. The room was very bright and there was a lot of activity. Victoria was lying on the bed with a protective shield in her chest area. There were many people in the room. The doctor and two other people were hovering over Victoria's belly. I was given a seat by her head, and I sat down. There seemed to be a lot of activity going on around Victoria's belly, and I couldn't see a thing. I stood up and peered over the protective barrier to see what was going on. The doctor had made an incision into Victoria's abdomen, and there was a lot of blood. I looked down at Victoria and asked her if she was okay. I had a mask on, so fortunately she could not see the look of horror on my face because they had just started doing the incision into her uterus. She had no idea of what I had just seen.

All of a sudden I saw James Michael in the doctor's hands. Shock came over me again, and I couldn't speak. One of the nurses took the camera from my hand and took a photograph of him for me. Jamie started to scream and wail, as a strong baby should. He looked so beautiful with the little hat that the nurses had put on his head. Before I could take in more detail of Jamie, Luke William was in the doctor's hands, and he too was shrieking at the top of his lungs. Eventually, I heard myself saying that I couldn't believe that my boys were here at last. There was such a lot of activity in the room. I didn't know what to do. Both Jamie and Luke had their own set of doctors and nurses taking care of them, and Victoria had her set taking care of her.

I peered over a nurse's shoulder and finally saw Jamie being weighed and measured, and then swaddled. They put Jamie in my arms, and I brought him over to Victoria. Victoria had tears of joy running down her face, and so did I. I was so happy. Luke was weighed, measured, and swaddled, and then handed to me. Again I went over to Victoria to show her our bundles of joy. There wasn't a dry eye in the room. It was such a magical moment, one that I will never forget. Again a nurse took the camera and snapped a photograph of me, with my bundles of joy in my arms.

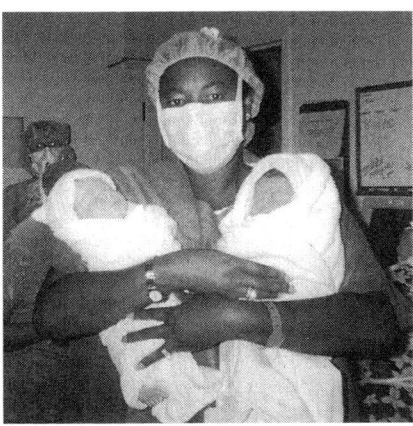

At last. I was a mother now!

My boys were born at thirty-six weeks. James Michael was born on August 29, 2001, at 5:45 PM. He weighed six pounds and fifteen ounces, and measured nineteen and a half inches long. Luke William was born at 5:47 PM, and he weighed five pounds and measured seventeen-and-a-half inches long. The nurses let me hold my babies for a while before they wheeled them off to the nursery. While I was holding both of my babies I did not have a free hand, and I wondered how on earth I would feed them both.

I telephoned my father to tell him that he had two healthy grandchildren. I also called my dear friend Fiona in the UK to tell her our happy news. By the time I got around to calling her it was about 3 AM, her time, because the UK is eight hours ahead of California. She told me beforehand that she did not mind what time of day or night it was when I called. It was great to share the news with her.

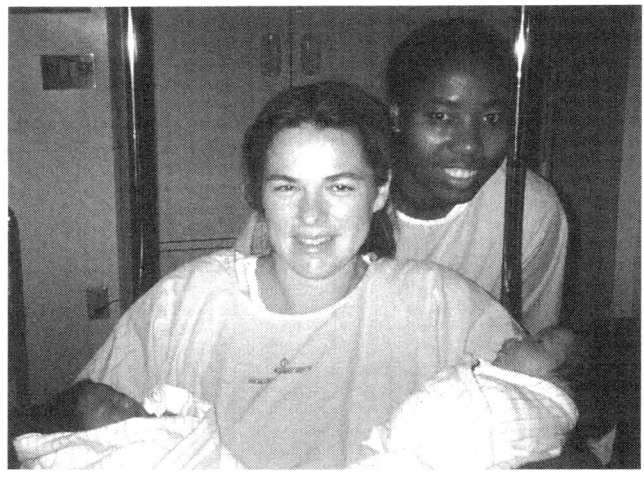

Victoria holding our bundles of joy, Luke and Jamie.

I then went over to see Victoria. She looked really good after the birth, although she was in a little pain. My brother Clive arrived, and he was able to see his new nephews before they went to the nursery. We stayed with Victoria for a while, and then we went over to the nursery to peer through the glass. My boys were so tiny and so beautiful. I was on cloud nine, and in disbelief. My boys were perfect, and I could not stop staring at them. At last my family was here. Craig would be arriving the next day, and then our family would be complete.

After we had peered through the glass for more than an hour, a nurse came over to us and said that my brother and I could go into the nursery to look at my sons. I was so grateful to her, because I desperately wanted to be with them. They were both given vitamin K shots, and they screamed so loud that I thought I would faint. I was so upset for them that I started to cry, too. My boys were in pain, and I really felt it myself.

While we were staring at Jamie and taking in every inch of his body, a nurse came over to us and announced that Luke was breathing rapidly, and that she was going to call the doctor. My immediate thought was that something terrible was going to happen next. I wanted to hold Luke, but we were asked to leave the room while the doctor came and examined him. After the examination, the doctor came out to speak to us and said that Luke would have to go to the neonatal intensive care unit (NICU) because his breathing was rapid. This was a condition known as *tachypnea*. He then told us that he should be okay to go home in a few days, but they wanted to monitor him closely. I started to worry again because the NICU was known for having very sick babies, and so Luke must have been very sick. I had never heard of tachypnea before, and it sounded really serious. When Luke was taken to the NICU, the nurses and doctors assured me that they just wanted to monitor his breathing.

With a very heavy heart I went back to the nursery to see Jamie. He was able to stay in the nursery because he was fine. I started talking to him, and I told him that I was his mother. I asked him if he remembered my voice. I told him that we had waited for such a long time to see him, and I was happy that he finally came. He seemed to be looking at me, and I was sure that he knew who I was.

Once Luke had settled into the NICU, I was allowed to visit him. I had to scrub each arm and hand for three minutes with a special soap and brush, so I could be sterile and free of germs before I entered the NICU. I scrubbed very carefully, because I did not want to contaminate the area. I also had to wear a gown. The nurse showed me where Luke was, and I gingerly walked up to him. He was so tiny and beautiful. He was lying in an incubator with a tiny diaper on. He was moving his arms and legs around, and I could see his little chest rising and falling. I could not take my eyes from him. He was so fragile, and I was afraid to touch him. Everyone assured me that he was fine, so after a while I left Luke in the NICU.

I went to say good night to Jamie, who was in the nursery, and then went back to the delivery ward to say goodnight to Victoria, and to thank her again. My brother and I went back to his house. I was exhausted and very worried about Luke. I telephoned Craig to tell him the doctors said that Luke needed to stay in the NICU, but that he should be fine in a day or two. Craig was also very worried. He felt so far away. He would be arriving the next day, and then we would both go to the NICU and see Luke together.

I woke up at about 6:00 the following morning, and I went straight over to see Victoria. I wondered if I was too early for visiting time, but the nurse did not say anything about my early arrival. Victoria looked very gray, and she was in a great deal of pain. She had never had surgery before, and she was having a lot of discomfort. I felt really guilty again. She went through all of this for us to have our babies. I still couldn't believe she had done this for us.

Breastfeeding encourages the uterus to contract to prevent post delivery bleeding. Because Victoria was not going to breastfeed, the nurses came in to massage Victoria's uterus to help it to contract. She let out a sound that I had never heard before. She was in a great deal of pain. I had to leave the room briefly to keep from throwing myself at Victoria's feet and begging her forgiveness for causing all this pain. Once the nurses had finished their duties, I gingerly walked back into the room. Victoria did not complain about the pain, and I don't know what I would have done if she did.

Jamie was brought to Victoria's room and placed in my arms. He was so beautiful. I will never forget his face that morning. I handed him to Victoria so that she could hold him, too. After a short while he started to cry, so Victoria handed him back to me. We decided that he was hungry. I had been given supplies by the nurses and told how to feed him. He didn't have any problems sucking, and he drank a great deal.

Eventually Craig arrived and came straight over and took Jamie from my arms. He held him as though he'd held him many times before. "Where have you been?" he asked. "We've been waiting for you." What a beautiful moment that was. Craig held him until Jamie fell asleep in his arms. We put him back in the little cot next to Victoria's bed and went over to see Luke in the NICU.

Craig and I scrubbed ourselves for three minutes as directed and put on our paper overalls. We went over to where Luke lay. He was doing very well, although we could still see his tiny chest rising and falling quite distinctly. We were able to stay with him for a long time. The nurses were very kind and caring, and they encouraged me to bond with my baby. I sat in the chair next to his incubator, and the nurse took Luke out of the incubator and handed him to me. She told me that I should open up my shirt and let Luke lie on my chest, skin to skin, so that he would be warm and could listen to my heart beat. He was so tiny, and I was afraid that I would drop him. At last I could bond with my baby! I was very happy.

I tried to feed Luke with a bottle, but I just couldn't do it properly. He would not swallow the milk. He didn't seem to know what to do with the nipple when it was placed in his mouth. This, of course, was very upsetting to me, because I now worried that he would not eat. A very sympathetic nurse came over to me and explained that some newborns have a problem sucking, so she told me to stroke his throat when I put the nipple in his mouth. No sooner had I started to do this, he started to suck. After a short while he had a very strong suction.

Craig wanted to feed him, too. I thought that he might have been scared, as I was, because Luke was so small, but he wasn't. I was so amazed by Craig. I thought that he might be clumsy with our babies, but he was not at all. It was as though he had been feeding babies for a very long time. He was a natural.

The nurses showed us how to bathe and clothe Luke. They also showed us how to change his diaper. We found these nurses to be particularly kind and caring.

Jamie was discharged from the hospital the next day, and we immediately took him over to the NICU to see his brother. When we arrived, we were told that we were not allowed to bring Jamie into the NICU because of germs, so Craig and I took turns seeing Luke while the other stayed with Jamie. We spent many hours in the family area of the NICU and by Luke's bedside. He was improving every day. What beautiful babies we now had to call our own.

When we got back to Victoria's house that night, Marcus and Chloe, Victoria's children, made such a fuss over Jamie. He was such a precious bundle of joy. When we went to bed that night, Craig and I placed Jamie between us. We did not sleep a wink, because we kept checking to see if he was still breathing. The only times we knew for certain that he was breathing were when he was awake and when he was feeding. We were so concerned about our precious gift. In the end, we decided to take turns so that maybe we would get at least an hour of sleep each, but we still didn't fall asleep. By the nightlight we could see his beautiful face, and we both just stared at him until it was time to get up the next morning.

Victoria was discharged from the hospital the next day and was starting to get some color in her cheeks. I was happy to see that she was doing so well, and I felt fractionally less guilty than I did the day before. She was happy to be back at home in her own environment.

On September 2, 2001, Luke was finally discharged, and we were really happy to have our family together. Jamie and Luke were a little yellow with jaundice, so we were instructed to put them in the sunlight inside the house, and we did so at every opportunity we had. We had put little socks on them, and one of the times when they were in the sun Luke sneezed, and one of his socks came off. He was so tiny, and his skin appeared to be too big for him. We all had a good laugh about it, and we loved him even more. We loved the sounds and the movements they made. When they were hungry, we fed them, and we changed them and laid them down to sleep. We would give Victoria one of our babies to hold, and she would stare at them just as much as we did when we held them.

Victoria and Clive's neighbors came over to see our boys and brought beautiful gifts for them. They had been incredibly kind and supportive of Victoria while she was pregnant. On one of the evenings when we came home from the hospital after the birth, a neighbor had cooked a meal for us all. That was very generous and timely, because we had not thought about food until we got home. It was great that dinner was there ready and waiting for us.

We took our boys to a pediatrician to make sure that they would be okay to fly back home with us to New Jersey. He gave them a clean bill of health, and when we got back to Clive and Victoria's house we arranged our flight to go home.

Part VI
Going Home

16

Our Journey Home

We stayed with Clive and Victoria for another week, and then Craig, Jamie, Luke, and I left to go home on September 9, 2001, to start our family life together. Our beautiful boys were eleven days old and a joy to behold. We decided to go to the airport in style, so we hired a limousine to take us there. We strapped the baby carriers into the seats and then said our goodbyes. Victoria had tears in her eyes, and so did I. She had been so wonderful to do this for us, and I didn't quite know how to thank her. I hugged Clive and Victoria, and again I thanked them both with all my heart. We said goodbye to Marcus and Chloe and got into our limousine. As we started down the road, we waved until we couldn't see them anymore. I was really sad to leave them all behind, but I was happy to be starting a life together with my new family.

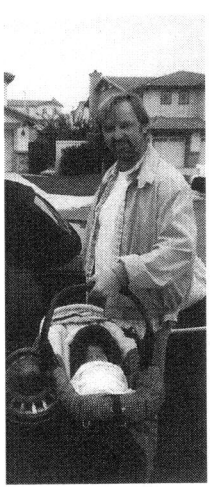

Luke with his proud dad, Craig, before we set off for the airport.

When we arrived at the airport, there were many smiling faces. Babies really do make people smile. Many people came up to us and asked how old they were. Fortunately, no one came too close to our boys. I was feeling very protective of them, and I didn't want anyone to touch them. Many times in the previous months I had worried that my maternal instinct would not start because I hadn't given birth to my sons. I needn't have worried. Even though they were only eleven days old, I felt they had always been with us.

The flight attendants were incredibly helpful and supportive throughout our journey home. They gave us everything we needed. We each held a baby on our lap, and again we stared at them to make sure that they were breathing.

When we arrived at Newark airport we were met by one of our neighbors, who had come to help us with our luggage. It was a great help, because we were really loaded up with babies, bags, bottles, diapers, wipes, and so forth. Craig and I didn't have a free hand between us.

As we drove down toward our house, we saw that our neighbors Mia and Hannah had put a "Welcome Home" banner on our garage door and tied balloons to our mailbox. What a lovely surprise that was. Not only that, they had filled our fridge with essentials. It truly was wonderful. Babies do bring out the best in people!

17

Family Life

I knew that the first couple of months were going to be difficult but I had no idea how difficult that time would actually be. We were constantly tired and felt that we were not doing things right because our babies were crying all the time. Craig had to go to work after a couple of weeks of their birth and he was exhausted. I felt very inadequate and upset all the time because nothing I did seemed to settle them.

We would feed one baby and settle him and then the other baby would start crying and demand to be fed. It seemed that feeding, changing and settling were going on for 24 hours a day with no breaks in between. Fortunately I remembered a book that I had read before our boys were born. The book said that we should try to put our babies on the same feeding schedule and they would, hopefully, feed, and sleep at the same time so that we could sleep while they were sleeping. We decided to give it a try. It took some time because one would want to feed and the other didn't. Eventually we managed to get them on more or less the same schedule.

When Jamie woke up we would wake Luke and try to feed them at the same time. I would prop them up on cushions and then feed them. Luke would take his time drinking his formula because he never seemed to be as hungry as Jamie.

Craig and I came up with a routine where only one of us would be awake at night. When Craig came home from work, I would go to sleep and he would take care of our babies. He would wake me up at midnight and then go to sleep. I would look after our boys during the night until about 5 AM and then Craig would take over and I would go to sleep until he was ready to go to work. He would wake me up just before he left for work. He would try to catch up on some of his missed sleep by falling asleep on the train.

This routine really was a shock to our systems at first but we found it to be the best way to manage the first couple of months. We learned to treasure the moments when we would all be asleep at the same time.

Jamie was the first one to sleep for five hours at night and this was heaven. Eventually Luke caught up and was able to sleep for almost five hours. This meant that

Craig and I could both have a block of at least four hours sleep before I would have to get up again.

Craig would prepare the bottles of milk for the next day. Our fridge was filled with bottles of formula. I read an article that said that the microwave should not be used to heat formula because of hot spots and scalding. I decided that I would boil water, pour it into a bowl, and then stand the bottles in the bowl of hot water. This would take a few minutes to heat the formula and often I would forget that I had bottles standing in hot water and by the time I remembered, the formula would be too hot for the babies to drink! Eventually, I gave in and decided to use the microwave which worked really well because the milk would be warm after only waiting for 20 seconds. I would shake the bottle vigorously to make sure there were no hot spots.

Even though the first couple of months were really hard, it was wonderful to have our boys in our home. Our house was alive with babies and musical toys. Life took on a new meaning now. We both had a sense of purpose and responsibility. We treasured our boys in every way. Craig would videotape our boys every time they moved. He would also take photographs at every opportunity.

Jamie and Luke had completely different personalities from day one. Jamie was a lot more vocal and Luke was always looking around to see what was going on. They really were perfect in every way. We enjoyed the sounds they made, their smell, and their movements. When they discovered they had hands Craig videotaped this monumental occasion. Jamie would stare at his hands for hours.

At the end of the day I would sit in the rocker and rock gently with them both in my arms until we all fell asleep.

Victoria and Clive—thank you both for your extreme generosity and kindness.

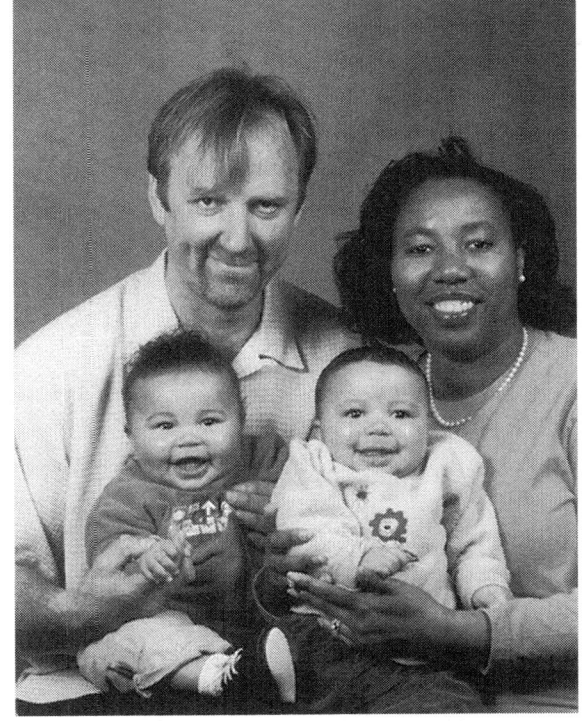

Jamie, Luke, Craig, and Sandra. At last our family was complete.

PART VII
Update

18
Our Boys Today

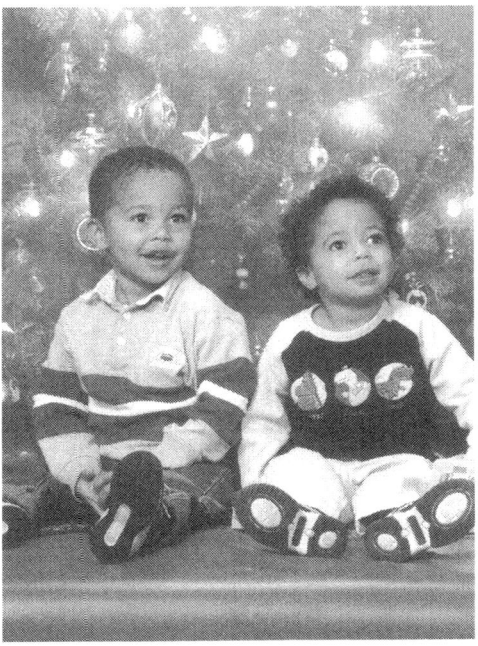

Jamie and Luke

Today Jamie and Luke are healthy three and a half-year-old boys. They both love to ride their bicycles. Jamie loves books and puzzles and Luke loves his cuddly toy puppy and trains.

Our friendship with Clive and Victoria has remained strong, if not stronger than it was before the surrogacy. A fear I had throughout our journey was that something would happen that would destroy our relationship and, thankfully, that did not happen at all.

Victoria is Jamie's and Luke's special aunty and, when they are not busy playing, they love to talk to her on the telephone.

Over the past three and a half years, I have told our boys many times that we wanted them very much, but my tummy was broken, and so Victoria offered to carry them in her tummy for us. Now that they are three and a half, they understand a lot more than they did the last time I told them this. This time Luke asked, "Is your tummy still broken, Mommy?" I said yes. "Can I kiss it better?" Jamie asked. They both kissed my tummy better, while tears of happiness rolled down my face.

"Intended Parents: Miracles Do Happen"

Afterword

While going through the process of surrogacy I founded the agency Intended Parents.com Inc and Web site www.intendedparents.com to help other intended parents go through the process of surrogacy. www.intendedparents.com is a multi-faceted website offering a wealth of information and support for those embarking on surrogacy as a way to create or expand their families. Intended Parents.com Inc is a full-service agency, matching surrogate mothers and egg donors with intended parents worldwide. I can be contacted via e-mail at Sandra@intendedparents.com

978-0-595-35528-0
0-595-35528-5

Made in the USA
Lexington, KY
30 September 2016